BOWEN UNRAVELLED

BOWEN UNRAVELLED

A JOURNEY INTO THE FASCIAL UNDERSTANDING OF THE BOWEN TECHNIQUE

JULIAN BAKER

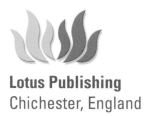

Lotus Publishing
Chichester, England

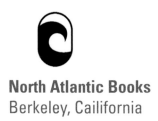

North Atlantic Books
Berkeley, Cailifornia

First published in 2013 by

Lotus Publishing

Apple Tree Cottage, Inlands Road, Nutbourne, Chichester, PO18 8RJ and

North Atlantic Books

P. O.Box 12327

Berkeley, California 94712

Drawings Amanda Williams and Emily Evans
Photographs Primal Pictures and Gil Hedley
Text Design Simon Hempsell
Cover Design Paula Morrison
Printed and Bound in Singapore by Tien Wah Press

MEDICAL DISCLAIMER

The following information is intended for general information purposes only. Individuals should always see their health care provider before administering any suggestions made in this book. Any application of the material set forth in the following pages is at the reader's discretion and is his or her sole responsibility.

Bowen Unravelled: A Journey into the Fascial Understanding of the Bowen Technique is sponsored by the Society for the Study of Native Arts and Sciences, a nonprofit educational corporation whose goals are to develop an educational and cross-cultural perspective linking various scientific, social, and artistic fields; to nurture a holistic view of arts, sciences, humanities, and healing; and to publish and distribute literature on the relationship of mind, body, and nature.

British Library Cataloguing-in-Publication Data

A CIP record for this book is available from the British Library

ISBN 978 1 905367 40 5 (Lotus Publishing)

ISBN 978 1 58394 765 4 (North Atlantic Books)

Library of Congress Cataloging-in-Publication Data

Baker, Julian, 1962- author.

 Bowen unravelled : a journey into the fascial understanding of the

Bowen technique / Julian Baker.

    p. ; cm.

Includes bibliographical references.

ISBN 978-1-58394-765-4 I. Title.

[DNLM: 1. Massage. 2. Fascia. 3. Physical Therapy Modalities. WB537]

RM721

615.8'22--dc23

                    2013022828

CONTENTS

INTRODUCTION 7

1 FASCIA 11

2 ANATOMY: NEW LAMPS FOR OLD 17

3 TOM BOWEN, 1916–1982 25

4 THE BOWEN MOVE 33

5 PAGE ONE 45

6 PAGE TWO 51

7 PAGE THREE 57

8 ANKLE 63

9 BREAST 69

10 COCCYX 73

11 DIAPHRAGM AND RESPIRATORY SYSTEM 81

12 ELBOW 89

13 HAMSTRINGS 95

14 KIDNEY 103

15 KNEE 107

16 PELVIS 113

17 SHOULDER 129

18 TEMPOROMANDIBULAR JOINT 139

19 GETTING 'THEM' BETTER: THE OUTCOME PARADIGM 147

20 REASONS WHY BOWEN WORKS: PLACEBO EFFECT? 151

21 EFFECTIVE NOTE-TAKING: CLIENT AND THERAPIST OBSERVATION AND MARKERS 153

22 CONCLUSIONS 159

RESOURCES 161

INDEX 163

DEDICATION
To Jane

ACKNOWLEDGEMENTS

For the last few years I have had the enormous good fortune to be able to conduct fascial dissections with the kind permission of Imperial College of Medicine, under the watchful and supportive eye of Professor Ceri Davies and the ever-patient manager of the human anatomy unit, Rachael Waddington. Their help, advice and friendship has been invaluable and many of the images of dissections in this book appear by kind permission of the Human Anatomy Department, Imperial College of Medicine, London.

I am indebted also to the incredible kindness of the unnamed donors and their families, whose incredible gift of their forms makes the understanding of techniques such as Bowen, possible. The preparation of these forms is an art in itself and Lee Dennis is, in my view, the undisputed master. His skill, endless assistance and encouragement over the past few years has made the journey into dissection a lot easier than it could have been and I am eternally grateful.

To those too many to mention who have challenged me, supported me, fought me and bought me coffee, I thank you and hope that these pages will not let you down.

INTRODUCTION

The Bowen Technique was first taught in the UK in 1993 and since then has become well established in the mindset of complementary therapists all over the UK and the rest of Europe. When I arrived back in the UK in 1992 after living in Australia for five years, I was convinced that the revelation of Bowen would change the way in which we think of and treat the body. This was a little ambitious to say the least, and two hard years of slog followed. In spite of two courses being run in 1993, interest was poor and the fervour of conviction did little to fan the flames of interest. The saving grace was an article by Jane Alexander in the *Daily Mail* in April 1994: this prompted an enormous response, with over ten thousand people contacting us to find out about treatment or training.

My full-time career in the Bowen Technique had started, and has continued unabated ever since. In 1998 my partner, Louise Atwill, and I parted company with the people I had been working with; equipped with new-found freedoms, I began to move Bowen in a different direction. Previously the technique had been marketed to the alternative end of the therapy market, with little emphasis on the anatomical reasoning or scientific understanding of how Bowen might be working. While continuing to teach the original form of the technique, I decided to target the primary health care sector, attempting to inform chartered physiotherapists and medical professionals of the role that Bowen might be able to play. Alongside this, I needed to explore in more depth the anatomy of the body, and question some of the conclusions that were being drawn about what was or was not happening, and what was also possible.

In 1999 I met Hans Thijssen, a remarkable bodyworker and intuitive therapist, who introduced me to the role that fascia played in the workings of the body and in particular to the way that physical therapy might affect this remarkable material. When one starts down a particular path it is sometimes difficult to see how or where the twists and turns will take you, and I can say with confidence that some key people have made a difference to how my understanding has changed and continues to evolve. Hans was key in what was to follow.

In 2002 Michelle Marr, a neurophysiotherapist, contacted me. She wanted to use Bowen to explore how it might affect hamstring flexibility, and, as part of her MSc, designed the first thorough examination of the effects of Bowen. Her immense knowledge and perfect power of explanation has inspired me continuously ever since; our joint explorations into fascia and connective tissue – through dissection, reading and lots of heated debate – has moved me on, both personally and intellectually, in ways I could never have imagined. I can honestly say I would not be where I am today without her.

More recently I have had the incredible good fortune to work with Gil Hedley, a mad professor if ever there was one. Gil divides his time between home educating his kids in Florida and flying around the USA (and once a year the UK), running the most incredibly inspirational dissection workshops, which show a different perspective on how and why the body does what it does. Gil demonstrates that the body comes in layers rather than parts, and his passion is to resist the established view and find a different way of looking both at the world and at the body. He is funny, warm and endearing to all he meets, and what he doesn't know about a body isn't worth knowing. No one who attends Gil's workshops can ever look at bodywork, the world or themselves in quite the same way–myself included. It was Gil who has inspired me on my journey into the dissection process and allowed me to find answers and find direction to my work and my place in the world. Being around Gil to me means laughter and joy and I value his continued friendship and counsel beyond measure.

Tom Myers, another inspiring character with whom I have had many discussions and debates, once said something along the lines of: "Every five years or so, you need to realise that everything you have done up until now is bullshit, throw it all away and start again." Tom was a good lesson in demonstrating that what might be insulting to one person is a challenge to another, and I am grateful for the fire he has lit under me.

Whilst I'm not about to dispense with both baby and bathwater, my shifts have been large and my leaps of faith larger. I am not an academic, and have no university education and indeed no academic qualifications. I left school at the age of 16 and became an apprentice chef, working my way through the sweaty ranks of various hellhole kitchens around London. Cooking is a tough game, but also an incredibly tactile and emotional environment. You get to feel what you are working with, and I am in no doubt that this was a strong grounding in being able later in life to feel textures altering under my hands when trying to change bodies. It also allowed me to approach anatomy and structural study side on, without having a formulated understanding or adherence to any one particular school of thought.

From my sometimes childlike perspective, the old and long-accepted paradigms didn't always make sense, and so I kept asking, 'Why?' We are often presented with facts that, it seems, we should accept at face value simply because 'that's how it is'. I challenge that view wherever it seems obvious that there is another way of thinking. Many people of a certain age will be told that there is nothing that can be done for their pains or conditions because 'it is your age'. Is this true? I doubt it.

My views and approaches over the years have, I am the first to admit, at times been confrontational and opinionated, and in my naïve desire to push my views, beliefs and theories forward I have probably offended and alienated some people. But I also hope that at the same time I have managed to cut through some of the more cloudy theories and put across ideas which have perhaps inspired and excited others. Time and obituaries will tell.

This book aims to clarify some of the myths and misconceptions that have arisen around the Bowen Technique over the years. At the same time, I hope to bring Bowen forward as one of the leading and most effective connective tissue therapies available. This can only be done by speaking the same language and using the same terms as are traditionally used by allopathic and complementary therapies the world over.

I welcome debate, discussion, argument and questioning. These have been lacking in the field of complementary medicine for too long, and we need to be constantly self-evaluating, growing and questioning our own acceptance of what we do, if we are ever to be taken seriously. I am tired of endlessly seeing valid and effective therapeutic approaches ridiculed and belittled, simply because they do not conform to an established perspective. I welcome the chance to promote complementary therapy in general, and Bowen in particular, as a viable and useful addition to the health and wellbeing of the country.

The views I express here are very much my own and do not necessarily represent anyone else I am associated with or work with. I accept that for the most part I am probably wrong, and will take every opportunity to find out just how wrong I am in order to adjust my perspective. Each day is a new opportunity to change and learn.

Mahatma Gandhi was once asked a question about some matter, to which he gave a clear and direct answer. The following day he was asked virtually the same question and gave an entirely different answer. Those present the previous day picked him up on this: "Yesterday, Gandhiji, you were asked the same question and gave a completely different reply." His response, inspirational and a demonstration of wisdom, was simple: "Yes, that is true, but today I am better informed."

Come the time that better information lands in my lap, I will put pen to paper again. Until then, please accept this humble offering in the spirit in which it is intended.

CHAPTER 1

Fascia

For the purposes of this discussion, it should be made clear that, whilst all fascia is connective tissue, not all connective tissue is fascia. The different types of fascia include cartilage, tendon, adipose tissue, bone and even blood. In the field of conventional medicine, connective tissue – be it fascia or any of the others mentioned – has had little in the way of attention. It is considered to be a supporting or filling structure that is responsible for binding and cementing, but with no other function or purpose. Yet there are strong views that suggest otherwise. Théophile de Bordeu, an 18th-century physician, recognised that connective tissues carried out regenerative functions for certain organs and acted as circulatory and nervous systems.

Connective tissue is the only tissue that has contact with every part of the body and does exactly what it says on the tin – it connects! For this reason it is a system which we should take a great deal of notice of. In addition, within the functional role of connective tissue, there is a function of cleansing and washing. "Everything that comes out of the blood takes a somewhat complicated route through the connective tissue to the parenchymal (thin walled cells) and then into the lymph system" (Pischinger 2007).

SKIN AND SUPERFICIAL FASCIA

I put these two structures together in one title from the perspective of a bodyworker or therapist rather than from that of an anatomist. There is plenty of study material available about the skin, and even some about the superficial fascia, but it is the relationship of these two materials that is of interest here.

The skin is the largest organ of the body and referred to by Deane Juhan as "the surface of the brain" (Juhan 2003). It quite literally breathes, and acts as an organ of waste removal, temperature control and infection protection. It is an emotional layer – a layer that allows us to react to the world around us and to feel good or bad. Something might make our skin 'crawl', or we might feel mentally and physically more balanced when the sun is on our skin. A continuous structure, the skin moves, distorts, grows and shrinks with us as we grow, and it reflects our health, our climate, our age, our wellbeing and even our emotional state. Have you ever blushed from embarrassment, sweated through fear or gone white with shock?

Attached to the skin in an intimate relationship is the underlying superficial fascia layer. This layer is often called the adipose (or subcutaneous) tissue, and, although containing the two types of adipose tissue, white and brown, it is also much more than just a fatty layer. The superficial layer gives us the springy feel to our bodies and acts as a huge shock absorber, as well as being a very important infection-fighting layer. Its ability to easily store fat is one of the reasons we experience obesity. However, this layer is also an endocrine organ, secreting hormones such as leptin (Kershaw and Flier 2004), which is involved in the regulation of metabolism and appetite, and resistin, increased levels of which are suspected to play a role in obesity and insulin resistance. In addition, cytokines – cells secreted by the immune system that regulate and control inflammation and emergency responses throughout the body – are stored in the adipose tissue. This means that the superficial fascia, as an adipose layer, has all the equipment it needs, not just to store energy, but also to communicate with all the other organs of the body, including the central nervous system (CNS). And we thought it was just fat!

The superficial fascia is a loose, areolar layer of tissue, having the appearance of bubble wrap when examined. You can push your fingers in between the loose pockets of fatty, yellow material and gently tease it apart. Yet, at the same time as being almost fluffy and flexible, it is incredibly strong and able to absorb large pressures placed upon it. If, for example, you were to press hard and quickly onto it, then the layers would close in on themselves just like bubble wrap, and protect the underlying tissues from penetration or heavy pressure.

This fascia is adhered to the skin in an intimate arrangement that defies manual separation: the only way to examine this layer away from the skin is to use a very sharp blade and forcibly take the layer and the skin apart. Once separated from the skin, the layer is still incredibly strong, dense and continuous; even prolonged and strenuous pulling will not rip the layer. As well as its ability to contain fat, the superficial fascia is also a layer of connective tissue – it is three-dimensional and, like the skin, sits in a continuous layer all over the body. The thickness of the fascia varies from a couple of millimetres to several centimetres, but it is always connected to skin at its outer surface. In much the same way that the skin is the interlocutor between the inside of the body and the outside world, the superficial layer is also acting on the internal organs. It is heavily supplied with blood and fluids from the rest of the body, and is perforated throughout its surface by blood vessels and nerve endings that reach through and terminate on the surface of the skin.

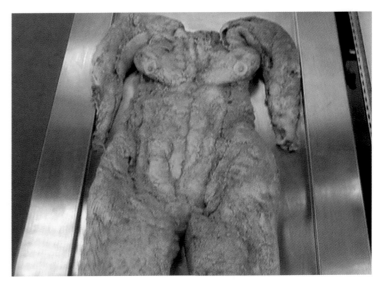

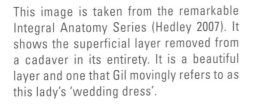
This image is taken from the remarkable Integral Anatomy Series (Hedley 2007). It shows the superficial layer removed from a cadaver in its entirety. It is a beautiful layer and one that Gil movingly refers to as this lady's 'wedding dress'.

The superficial layer is also a particularly poor conductor of heat, which means that it is very helpful in retaining the heat of the body and keeping us warm. So with all these useful qualities we have to wonder why we have such a poor relationship with it. The fatty layer that is our superficial fascia is often demonised. We are concerned about having less fat in and on our bodies, which is fine. But we also go to great lengths to lose weight and burn fat, seeing it as something to be excised, and even going to such extremes as liposuction and plastic surgery.

For the Bowen therapist, this is the layer with which we have most in common and through which we work when trying to reach into other structures of the body. It is always present underneath our hands; however much we wish to think about muscle, bone, deep fascia and so forth, it is this layer which is the translator of our touch to the deeper tissues beneath. When working, for instance, around the gluteal area, the depth of tissue is such that we are feeling a distant resonance of the gluteus maximus. Whilst we are able to define tension, tone and feeling of the underlying muscle, much of the quality of this palpatory sense will be subject to the sensitivity of how we approach the superficial fascia.

There are many deep tissue approaches in the world of bodywork, many of which involve the application of significant pressure to delve through the superficial tissues. However, it must be understood that, just because Bowen is a light touch, it is not excluded from the world of deep tissue. Indeed, you can access any areas of the body you wish from a Bowen perspective, but the factors that may prevent you from doing so are the tension you use and the way in which the superficial fascia responds to this tension.

If we work through the superficial layer with patience and a light touch, our ability to reach in, palpate and treat deeper tissues without creating pain or being invasive will be perfectly straightforward. My concerns arise from those therapists who think that in order to go deep you have to go in hard. This is, in my view, a huge mistake. Quite apart from being unpleasant and pointless, it also raises the real possibility of damage; there are many stories associated with therapists, even supposedly Bowen therapists, applying too much pressure, with too much tension, creating considerable increases in pain.

I need to make it very clear that, if you are creating a pain response as a regular feature of your Bowen work, you are incorrectly applying and understanding the principles of Bowen and need to reconsider both what you do and what you call it.

MUSCLE

In the world of sports injury, massage and most hands-on techniques, there is a very large focus on muscles and their movement. Much of the understanding of the individual components of a muscle is based upon the study of very trimmed meat, and on pictures which bear little resemblance to what the muscles actually look like.

We could say that there are over 800 muscles in the body, each having at least one nerve and a function; this fact has been defined and documented to the point that there can be no discussion or argument about it. My preference when discussing muscle is to refer not to muscles 'attaching' to this or that bone, but rather to use the word 'reference' instead. The use of 'reference' might appear semantic, yet this word implies continuity. It will help us to always understand that any given muscle is on its way somewhere and has come from somewhere else, and that these aspects should be considered when appraising muscular function.

It is, however, the connective element of what wraps around the muscles which creates more of an interest than anything else. If asked to put our hand on the abdomen, for instance, there is no doubt that we would all place it on the front of the body, somewhere around the navel. Yet there is as much, if not more, of an abdominal connection at the sacrum and lower back as there is in the small area at the front. It is at the back that all these groups come together to form one thickened and complex band, an understanding of which will be explored later on in this book.

So where does Bowen fit in with these myths of the body? Well, the beauty of Bowen is that you don't tend to, or shouldn't, look for sites of pain, but instead treat the body as a whole – hence the remarkable successes that we see, even with chronic, long-standing pain. Seven out of ten people in the UK will suffer from back pain at some time in their lives, and, according to the Office for National Statistics, the numbers are increasing. Over 100 million European citizens suffer from chronic musculoskeletal pain (CMP), though it remains undiagnosed in up to 40% of cases. In their guidelines, The National Institute for Clinical Excellence (NICE) state that the number of cases of low back pain are "only exceeded by mild to moderate mental health problems in the UK" (NICE 2009).

Traditional approaches for dealing with back pain are generally largely ineffective, and the treatment tends to focus on the area of pain. The NICE guidelines on the treatment of back pain run to over 250 pages, the conclusion being that there isn't much that can be done. We can put a man in space, but we can't sort out your back pain. Long-term non-specific back pain still remains a major cause of absence from work. I firmly believe that the major reason for this failure is a significant inability to grasp the concept of regarding the body as a connective tissue system: the back hurts because something else is happening to make it hurt. All the treatment in the world for the back will tend to have little effect in these instances.

Because Bowen works the upper, middle and lower back as part of its basic approach, it takes into account, often by luck rather than judgement, all the other areas that might affect the back. The connected nature of the deep fascia, which holds and binds the muscular network together, is not studied or noted in the teaching of anatomy to doctors. Also omitted from the teaching is the concept of how varied movements, postures, functions and habits help to lay down fascia and connective tissues, which in turn creates continued patterns and cycles of pain and a lack of effective function.

There are many books and Internet articles which will help you to learn how fascia is made and created, but I will attempt to give a simple precis of what fascia is, how it is made in our bodies and how it responds to the light touch that is, or should be, characteristic of the Bowen Technique.

COLLAGEN

The source of what we understand as deep fascia is collagen, exuded into the body by a cell called a fibroblast. There are dozens of types of collagen, and it is the most common protein in the body: it constitutes up to around 40% of all the protein in the human system.

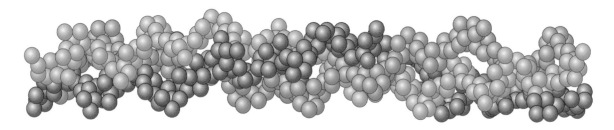

Collagen is the building block for our structures; where plants rely on cellulose to maintain their physical structure and shape, humans are similarly reliant on collagen. A large molecule, one of the largest in the body, collagen forms thick, twisted triple bands of densely packed fibres, which are then laid down all over the body to create fascia as well as a host of other tissues (see above). The cornea of the eye is collagen based, as are the strong ligaments around the knee. Wherever we see movement we see collagen, which is being produced all the time until the day we die.

In terms of the fascia, however, collagen has a particular role, and supports our frequent movements and postures. If we were to hold a certain position for any length of time, we would experience stiffness. This stiff feeling is the beginning of collagen fibres lining up and thickening. Continued lack of movement or stiffness may eventually lead to ossification and atrophy, and is characteristic of so many stooped and painful postures that we can see around us.

Fascia is laid down as a response to need, and it doesn't judge whether this is a good or a bad thing. Instead it lays down willingly according to what the body is asking for. A repetitive action will result in the creation by the fascia of the support around the muscle to fully integrate this action into the movement pattern of the individual. For instance, if you were a golfer trying to perfect a new stroke, you would need to repeat this movement thousands of times in order for your body to undertake this movement naturally and easily, and hopefully without having to think about it.

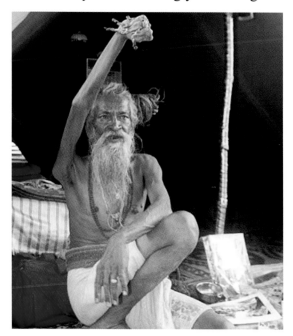

Amar Bharati has kept his arm raised as a tribute to Shiva for 38 years. We find this picture remarkable because it shows the stiffness that has come about as a result of this lack of movement. However the picture also shows what happens if you keep moving and don't keep a limb still. His hips and knees, used to years of squatting on the ground, show a remarkable level of flexibility for a man in his 70s. Keep moving and you'll keep moving. Rest and you rust!

Muscular movement is limited to the line of contraction that it takes to perform its function. The biceps contracts and flexes the arm. That's about the limit of its function; the triceps is then needed to contract in order for the arm to extend. Nevertheless the arm will flex and extend as part of a combination of thousands of movements every day, in conjunction with a lot of other movements around the body. As yet there is no science which looks at these relationships and how they fit together as part of the complex patterns of human functional movement.

If I raise my arm, I can allocate a series of muscles that will be responsible for this function. However, at the same time, I will need to stabilise my body in order to allow for a transference of weight and tension through my frame. The abdominal structures, and those surrounding the hip on the opposite side of the shoulder that is moving, will need to contract and become functional. If they don't, then the act of raising my arm will cause me to fall over. Is it my brain that is directing this stabilising and correcting pattern millions of times a day? It would seem to be something of a wasted resource if the brain were having to constantly adjust the body. Instead, we lay down fascia and supporting tissue to allow us to formulate habitual movement, with these tissues also serving to communicate with each other, forewarning, through tensional behaviours, what is about to happen. A spider's web of tensional information.

It stands to reason, therefore, that this web exists to aid human function and movement. It can also be utilised by the intuitive therapist, who can interpret tensions and patterns to assist the body on the road to self-correction. Perhaps we can even suggest that the connective tissue system is perhaps operating as an independent nervous system, working alongside the brain, but with some kind of functional autonomy. Certainly, the fascia operates in a way that current scientific thought hasn't yet fully explained, and it is probable that techniques such as Bowen will be seen in the future as the key to tapping into this newly discovered area of human function.

CHAPTER 2

Anatomy: New Lamps For Old

The traditional view of anatomy is arrived at simply because the body is divided in the same way that it has been for many hundreds of years. It is just the way it is. One anatomy book is going to be much like any other. Each muscle has a name, a function and nerves that innervate it. That's fine when dealing with structures in isolation, but when it comes to trying to understand how one bit of the body works in relation to another bit, the traditional anatomical view of the body has no answers. If anything, it actually denies relationships between far-off structures.

Modern medical study relies little on gross anatomy these days, and not at all on the wider relationships of systems to each other. Medical students obviously have to learn the systems of the body, the muscles and the bones, but there is no science that takes these students to one side at the end and explains how these things fit together. A medical condition has a symptom, which then has a diagnosis and finally a treatment. The idea of symptom, diagnosis and treatment is the holy trinity of modern medicine.

The concept of a relationship of structures in the process of cause and effect is alien to the allopathic model. How does one problem in the body impact on another area, or even create another problem? The diagnosis of a problem in the wrist might result in the treatment being surgery. Yet if the problem has originated from the neck, which in turn has come from a long-standing back pain, which originally was prompted by a torn ligament in the knee, and so on, then what hope is there for the wrist problem being solved?

All these answers are in the body, and a skilled reader and practitioner will pick these up through a combination of interview and observation. It is a skill which can be taught and learned in much the same way as a surgeon will learn his art. If the belief is that the knee cannot possibly lead to a wrist problem, and that it could in fact be true is considered to be 'alternative', 'weird' or just 'wrong', then there is little chance of the surgeon of the future changing his view that much. By understanding the body in terms of an interconnected tensional system, however, it becomes easy and logical to grasp the idea that strains, pressures, shortenings or pulls in one area will have a natural knock-on effect in other areas.

Tom Myer's view of the body as a tensional system has led to his very successful Anatomy Trains concept, something for which I have an enormous amount of respect. This system explains a complex series of lines of strain throughout the body, and allows the observer to try to pick up on where these strains might impact on the body's function. The lines aim to show the continuity that might exist through and around the body and impact on functional movement. I am often asked which book lays out the best principles of what I talk about in terms of function, and *Anatomy Trains* is as close as it gets and should be a feature of every therapist's book shelf. By breaking the body down into ways that a therapist might be able to spot functional imbalance Anatomy Trains helps to build a three dimensional view of the human form.

It is important to remember though, that these lines are simply a model from which to demonstrate the principle of continuity and don't exist by themselves. Learning the principles of the lines or similar approaches will discipline the therapist to stop looking at isolated pain presentations and instead allow a more global understanding of functional imbalance.

"Hold your theory lightly and your practice dearly." (Gil Hedley)

Modern medical thinking does not have an overall view of the body. A surgeon might know intimately the knee or hip that he is operating on, but has probably never taken a full body apart to see how that hip or knee relates to the other hip or knee, or indeed the shoulder or diaphragm. Yet these relationships do indeed exist in a very real and vital way. To ignore them is to end up with a small fraction of the full picture.

The integral view, however, is invariably dismissed as being 'alternative' or just wrong. My determination has therefore been to demonstrate the actual presence of these tissues and interfaces, in order to be able to state with absolute conviction that there is indeed a correlation between conditions of the face and problems in the lower back. With the power of this knowledge comes the ability to also demonstrate how these things manifest in posture and movement. With practice we can actually

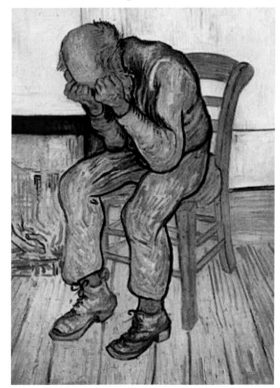

pick out pain from a client and show how this pain has developed and increased over a period of time. Tacked on to this approach is also the psychosocial element. If someone is in pain, how does their posture change? If someone is also emotionally or mentally challenged, how does this translate into the way they carry their body? (Levine 1997).

As we have seen, fascia changes and lays down patterns according to its given task. If the position of our head and neck is related to, or caused by, the emotional pattern that we have taken on, then we need to consider this as part of our treatment model. It is something that can naturally be experimented with. If we stand slouched forwards, arms dropped, head hanging down, with the back of the neck rounded,

Van Gogh's painting On the Threshold of Eternity is often used to demonstrate the physical face of despair experienced in depression. A similar result can be found by an Internet image search for depression.

and simply say out loud, "I feel really, really happy", then we are more likely to laugh. The posture in relation to the words seems ridiculous. If, in contrast, we stand up straight, push our chests out, lift our heads up and then say, "I feel depressed and unhappy", the same sense of contradiction arises.

This is a forced scenario, but the principle remains: we are in a symbiotic relationship with our emotions. We feel first, and react accordingly. Our feelings are enmeshed in our sense of self. We 'squirm' with embarrassment, or 'curl up' with it. We are 'sick' with fear, or 'paralysed' by nerves. When we are let down or disappointed, we might say we are 'gutted', reflecting our feelings inside.

The concepts of feeling and emotion have tended to be separated into distinct disciplines. We might see a doctor for a heart problem or a stomach problem, and a counsellor, psychotherapist or even psychiatrist for a mental disorder. Again the separation here is tenuous at best, and perhaps instead of asking how someone might feel, we might ask how and where someone is feeling. It is a subject which increasingly extends itself each time I touch on it, and one about which more writing might be called for in the future. But I do encourage all therapists to truly embrace the concept of the holistic approach, and include the nature and emotional state of the client. It is all too easy to 'medicalise' clients, trying to treat the condition rather than the person, and it is not a model I feel comfortable with.

ANATOMY: MORE TRADITION THAN SCIENCE

For many hundreds of years the study of anatomy has been driven by established approaches. It had its roots in the work of Galen, a Greek physician born in 129 AD, whose research and theories on human function were mainly based on the dissection of monkeys and pigs, as human dissection

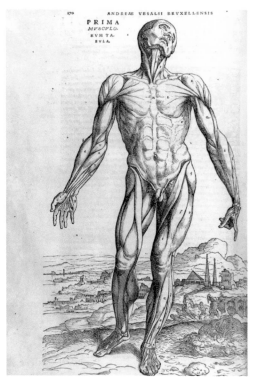

was forbidden by the Romans. In the mid-16th century, the Belgian physician Andreas Vesalius led the field in the use of human cadavers to study the workings of the body, and discovered that there was indeed quite a difference between humans and monkeys. He published pictures and descriptions of his dissections in *De Humani Corporis Fabrica* (see Saunders and O'Malley 1950).

The medical profession of the time was outraged, and Vesalius was even tried and condemned to death under the Spanish Inquisition, although his sentence was later commuted. Even then Vesalius stopped short of undermining the findings of Galen in respect of how blood circulates around the body. It was only in 1628 that the circulation of the blood with the heart as a pump was completely described in detail, by William Harvey, changing the views held to be true for over a thousand years. Still held as a central belief today, the theory of the brain controlling all muscle movement through the cranial and peripheral nervous systems

A plate from Andre Vesalius' De Humani Corporis Fabrica book (1543).

stemmed from experiments performed by Galen nearly two thousand years ago.

By the Georgian period, private anatomy colleges proliferated in London, and men such as John Hunter and his brother William fought tooth and nail to procure material to perform dissections and experiments, spawning the 'resurrectionists' (Moore 2006). These were men who, in the dead of night, would steal recently deceased bodies from graves and sell them to the anatomists, which led to pitched battles over opened graves. The scarcity of material created a lot of problems, and it was only by the introduction of the Anatomy Act of 1832 that the supply was regulated, and the atrocities of stealing the dead and murdering to order was brought under control.

The main body of influence in modern anatomical thinking, however, was Henry Gray, who, in 1858, published the first edition of what would become the seminal anatomical textbook for the next hundred years. Today, the 40th edition of Gray's Anatomy, which was published in 2010 (Drake, Vogl and Mitchell), is an updated version of the original. However, it is worth noting that, although modern anatomical thinking has changed and developed, it hasn't really become joined up.

Most medical students undertake very little in the way of dissection, and even the study of anatomy is limited to working with sections of tissue that have been prepared in a manner which has changed little in the past hundred years. Medicine is based on a segmented approach, and the understanding of the human body follows this thought process almost slavishly. Hence, newly qualified doctors will have had years of study under their belts, including an extensive knowledge of the various functions, workings and failings of the human body. They will have little or no understanding, however, as to how the functions are interlinked.

The preparation of tissue for study is carried out along fairly prescriptive lines, and the study itself is undertaken from texts and methods that haven't changed that much since the time of Vesalius. The human structure relies on its integral nature in order to move and function. Without the dependant relationships that characterise and underpin the human form, we would have no basis for studying the nervous or digestive systems. This lack of cohesive understanding, which could be considered to be a failing or a lack of integration within medicine, would be a sad omission were it not for a further tragedy. In the fields of manipulative medicine, complementary medicine, physiotherapy, chiropractic and osteopathy, the study of anatomy has tended to follow the same, somewhat incomplete, approach.

We study muscles and groups of muscles, and learn their actions and the nerves which supply them, but do not take into consideration the relationships that make them relevant to the rest of the body. We say that a biceps muscle flexes the arm, or that a deltoid is involved in abduction. Both statements are not untrue, but neither of them is exactly definitive when it comes to understanding function. In traditional anatomical thinking, I could reduce the lifting of my arm to a group of muscles based around the shoulder girdle, along with a few others around the chest and neck for good measure. If there is something causing me pain, or preventing me from performing this function, I will assume that the problem lies in the area of the presenting pain, and as a result will tend to treat this area as the problem.

In order for me to be able to lift my arm, however, a whole series of factors come into play. I need to be able to stabilise the rest of my body, as the act of lifting the arm will shift the weight around my centre of gravity. If the opposite side of my body is for some reason unable to support this shift, then I will need to compensate in another area. The result may well be that I lift or move my arm in a way that creates a conflict with what might be considered 'normal' movement. If there is a weakness associated with the compensating area, this could be the location of the problem, even though the pain or restriction is nowhere near this point. To most people it sounds pretty straightforward and obvious, and in many ways it is, but this element of simple cause and effect of movement is neglected and even denied by the traditional surgical segmented approach.

The myths of conventional anatomy are perpetuated by concepts which we hold true and dear, with an example of the skeleton being the best. We see skeletal images all over the place, and when walking into a classroom or anatomy lab we are faced with the ubiquitous presence of the wired skeleton with its rictus grin. The concept of a skeleton as a framework is an example of the problem we have. This is a created image, a myth, a sculpture – it bears no resemblance to anything we might see as truly existing within the human frame.

On the skeleton we can see two hundred or so bones joined together. It stands there as if, given some kind of brain and a malicious will, it could come to life and chase us, bony arms outstretched. The point is that the only reason it is standing there in the first place is because, much like the dead parrot of Monty Python fame, it is nailed there. If we took away the wires, screws, bolts and bits of plastic that hold the structure in place, it would simply fall apart, leaving a collection of bones on the floor. Each bone would have no relationship to any other bone, but would simply lie there as an individual piece of dog food. This relationship, or lack thereof, extends to every bone in the body, and begs the question of hard tissue adjustment techniques: what is it that they are adjusting exactly? Well, it can hardly be bone, which only leaves what is left – the soft tissues. Over to you, chiropractors!

The next stage is to add bits to the bones which will allow them to move around; it is at this point that we begin to introduce the muscles, ligaments and tendons which bind the bones in place and give the skeleton its mobility. The traditional view adds muscle and soft tissue in layers, creating the idea of there being certain groups that have certain functions. Whilst this is useful in terms of a learning tool, it is nevertheless far from definitive when we start to examine interconnected relationships. The learning of traditional anatomical models is helpful, if not essential, for the aspiring therapist. The problem arises when it is the sole element for studying the body. These models have been handed down by anatomy lecturers from generation to generation, with most lecturers never having seen a dissected human form, but teaching the inadequate knowledge from a book.

In illustrating parts of a body, there is a formula which is fairly rigid and which has been adhered to for a long time. However, the concept of there being more than one way to skin a cat extends upwards through the food chain. As Gil Hedley has aptly demonstrated, there are countless ways to dissect a body and demonstrate the individual nature of the human being (Hedley 2007). For example, there will be many who will be confident in their ability to identify the structure known as the iliotibial band (ITB) or tract, running down the lateral side of the leg to the tibia, and diverging into the quadriceps at the front and the glutes at the back. When running dissection courses, it is a particular pleasure of mine to ask students to find this tract, its beginning and its end. Because of the nature of the fascia that wraps itself around the leg, it quickly becomes evident that this is not a separate structure at all, but simply what is left when the dissector has trimmed away all the surrounding tissues.

The same holds with probably the majority of gross anatomical pictures, whether they be dissection pictures or illustrations. These pictures show what is left when everything else around it has been removed. The result is quite a distorted and sectional understanding of the human form, and one which has a lot missing. It begs the question that, if it is there on the human form on those around us, why is it so dismissed and diminished in the field of anatomical understanding?

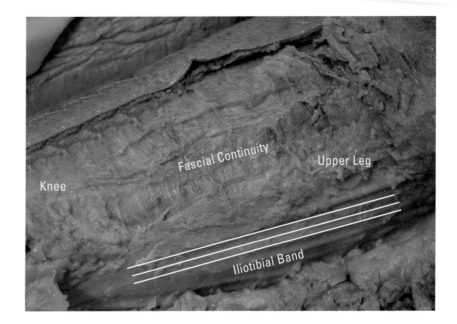

In this picture we can see what might clearly be described as the iliotibial band, but arising from it is the material normally cut away to leave the thickened band of fascia with which we are so familiar.

From my standpoint, the missing stuff is what I want to focus on. It is the superficial areas of the body that we, as hands-on therapists, need to focus on and understand, as it is these layers that we predominantly work on. Our study of deeper layers and muscle is of course useful, but the access to these structures is permitted and facilitated by the layers of skin, superficial fascia, deep fascia and connective tissues. If we don't see, feel and understand these layers, then any attempt to affect the deeper tissues is immediately arrested and compromised. It is also probable that, if treatments for conditions are devised around anatomy which is wrong, the treatments themselves might be questionable (Falvey et al. 2010).

The word 'superficial', however, conjures up a shallowness and lack of depth, leading to our immediate impulse to dismiss these layers as unimportant, or merely worthy of note in passing, on the way to something more interesting deep down. Yet no physical therapist ever touches muscle, tendon, bone or ligament, but merely feels these as reflections or projected images. If we understand this, then we must surely endeavour to understand the material through which we work and through which our deeper understanding is reflected.

The whole of what we are dealing with can be termed connective tissue in the broadest sense of the word, some of which is also called fascia. Does Bowen address bones? Certainly it does, as the act of releasing and unwinding the tensional relationships creates a potential for bony relationships to move and respond as they need to. There is rarely a need to crack or manipulate, and I would suggest that, if adjustment cannot be made or achieved through soft tissue release, it is unlikely to be achieved by manipulation or high-velocity thrust movements.

One muscle is connected to another muscle because of its fascial connections. Thus, for example, the pectoralis muscle is pretty much the same muscle as the deltoid muscle, so in order to separate these muscles you need to take a sharp knife and cut them. The fascia doesn't just surround the muscle – it surrounds all the spindles and the bundles of the muscle; it is also found around the bone in the form of a material that we call periosteum. It is the network that gives the body its integrity and ability to move around. Muscle is effectively pink and squishy, and made up of protein; without fascia it has no basis for movement, strength and connectivity.

"Muscle relies entirely for its integrity on the fascia that surrounds it." (Gil Hedley)

We need to understand that one can assign a function to a group of muscles: for instance, abduction of the shoulder (lifting of the arm sideways) will be assigned to muscles around the shoulder, such as the rotator cuff and so forth. Unfortunately, there are very few books on the market, if any, that will suggest or show the relationship between the shoulder and the abdominal muscles on the opposite side. Yet without the stabilisation, activation, and functional competence of this grouping, it will be impossible for me to lift my shoulder at all. I therefore need to understand the relationships of the structures rather than just the structures themselves. Bowen, either by design or by default, manages to address these relationships very effectively and practically, and this book will start to heighten your awareness of the existence and importance of these connections and relationships.

The bringing together of these systems has often been referred to as being holistic – a word which is rather used as an unpleasant stick with which to beat complementary therapy. However, it seems to be common sense to address the body as a complete unit and understand the relationships therein. The implications for this approach are enormous. As we have already discussed, the UK experiences epidemic levels of back pain; it is rarely treated or understood, and continues to be the cause of millions of lost working hours, and billions of pounds worth of treatment. Yet back pain is hardly ever just back pain – it can involve imbalances in the head, the knees and ankles, the pelvis and the abdomen, as well as having pathological causes.

As we start to move towards a greater understanding of the new anatomy, we will perhaps develop a wider acceptance of the whole-body model. It takes time, research, commitment and conviction, and it won't happen overnight. As was once said: "You can't stop a liner with a speedboat turn!" The ability of the body to change is reflected by the fact that collagen represents something in the region of 40% of all proteins in the body. Collagen is to humans what cellulose is to plants; it is the structural building block for movement and function, but at the same time it is also the building block for restrictions, calcifications and what we call our ageing process.

We continue to make collagen every day until the day we die; it is laid down in fascial tissues according to our movements, jobs, sports, injuries and so forth. Collagen is laid down in strong spiral units: each collagen fibril is a triple helix – three strands wound around each other in a tight spiral, banding together with other spirals to form structures and fascia having the strength of steel wire. It is these patterns that give us our postures, movement patterns, and even our habits, and in turn largely determine the way that muscle, and subsequently our whole body, moves. Spirals are the new model!

The behaviour of the superficial fascia in lots of environments begs the question whether the move might in some way create a soliton wave effect. Soliton waves were first described by the Naval engineer John Scott Russell in 1834. He saw a barge being pulled by a horse stop suddenly, and the wave that was at the prow continued unabated for quite a long way. He followed this wave for some distance and, after recreating the wave in his own laboratory, named it the 'Wave of Translation'. The theory of the soliton is used in the physics of fluid dynamics and aerodynamics, and it is possible that it could be a way of explaining the flow of a continuous wave-like energy through the body following a Bowen move. It's certainly a perfect image and explanation, and entirely possible in terms of energetic and fluid movement. Whether it fully explains how Bowen works is another matter.

Piezoelectricity is another word often mentioned in debates on tissue manipulation. Is the superficial fascia, the adipose layer, a piezoelectric layer? The word 'piezo' means to press or squeeze, and piezoelectricity is the energetic charge that builds up in certain materials in response to mechanical pressure. Hooke's law can perhaps help us to understand how the properties of deep fascia compare to those of a spring. The law says that the extension of a spring is directly proportional to the load applied to it. If we apply this law to the idea of potential energy being applied to a coiled spring, then we can understand that deep fascia can operate as a highly energetic structure and therefore a communicator. When we press onto a coiled, spring-like structure, there will be a recoil. This will come from the existing energy stored in the structure itself, known as its potential elastic energy, in addition to the pressure, or load, applied by the therapist – something which is harder to measure. If an attempt is made to apply a pressure that is equal to the tension in the tissues, then it will be the fascial structure itself which is going to be responsible for the change and release. In deep fascia, this change and energetic release can take place over a long period of time, hence the need to allow plenty of breaks and to not go in with too much pressure. It's not about the therapist!

In areas where the fascia is thickened, it seems reasonable to assume that the energetic potential is higher, meaning that 'stiffness', in spite of lack of apparent movement, might implicate an energetic concentration. Unfortunately, discussions such as this tend to be filled with maybes and perhaps, as we are very much in the field of relative ignorance. I read avidly the various proposals and ideas that come up to explain a Bowen move, but for the most part I have to admit that I am not a physicist or a mathematician and accept the limitations of my thought process. In all of this is the neural response that has to interpret any degree of energetic input coming from the range of mechanoreceptors in the skin.

Physics deals with constants and can define mathematically what it wants to demonstrate. The human form has always refused to conform to certainty, death aside, and I think it will be a long time before we can be certain of what is happening to us most of the time. To some this might seem a bit of a let down. How can we proclaim the effects of Bowen when we don't know precisely how it works? In reality, if we waited to know how things worked we'd get nowhere.

The miracle of human conception is still a complete mystery to the world. An egg is fertilised, and the woman's body then allows alien cells to proliferate. Not only does she allow this, but her body actively encourages it and provides a safe, nurturing environment for the embryo to grow, in direct defiance of all the laws of the immune system. Indeed, if this nut could be cracked, it would be a turning point for immune illnesses. The world of surgery owes its existence to the anaesthetist, who, if questioned carefully, will give you very convincing theory on how an anaesthetic works. In truth, he or she has no idea, but the theory will do for now. What is important is that we keep searching for ideas and thoughts, demonstrate clearly what is happening as being effective, and keep an open mind.

CHAPTER 3

Tom Bowen, 1916-1982

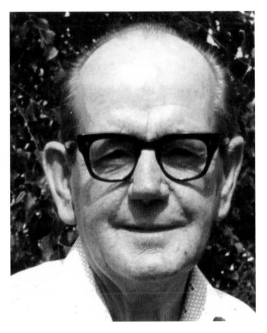

Tom Bowen.

A book about the Bowen Technique would not be complete without at least some reference to the man who gave the technique its name. There is plenty of information available in the public domain regarding the life and times of Tom Bowen, and this book does not pretend to be about the man himself. If truth be told, the book might not really even be about his technique, original or otherwise. Many people lay claim to his work and discuss whether their work is more like his, or whether they are being truer to what he was doing.

Much of the discussion regarding Tom Bowen in relation to current thinking is, without seeming or wanting to appear disrespectful, somewhat irrelevant now, many years after his death. Bowen referred to himself as an osteopath, yet had no training or background to back this title up. He did apply to go onto the osteopathic register in 1981 but was turned down for this very reason. His work was based on intuition, a clear understanding of the true nature of what the client was presenting with, and obvious self-belief in the restricted powers of the human body.

Bowen claimed to be performing up to 13,000 treatments a year, with most of them being first or second treatments. His waiting room was characterised by a number system. With no set appointments, people arriving would take a number from the board and wait to be seen. He described his ability as a 'gift from God', but it is likely he picked up hints and tips as he went along, especially from those around him to whom he was showing his method. Similarly, he never tried to explain how or why his method worked or what the principles were. Perhaps the level of understanding and vocabulary were not at his command, but perhaps also he was content to simply work with as many people as possible and not question how or why.

It is worth putting his life and work in context, giving some comparisons from today. When Bowen started working, there was no established complementary therapy industry, and he was not some kind of mystical new-age guru. He was a true Australian bloke who liked a smoke, a drink, his cricket and sports in general. Much as some people would like to believe, he had no contact with Aboriginal culture, Asian culture or anything else that would fit our ideas today. He played in the Salvation Army band, worked as a general hand at the local cement works and cared for his family.

His healing career, if you can call it that, took off purely and simply because of demand: people were in pain and he could help them. Stories abound of the remarkable things that happened in his clinics, but Bowen never took personal credit or created an image for himself. He never even called his technique 'the Bowen Technique' – he was just the bloke that fixed people up.

He taught a number of people, all men, over the years, having them come and observe his work for one morning a week. All of these men have varying interpretations of what they saw. Perhaps he showed them different things, or perhaps they understood differently what they saw, according to their own approaches. In any case it is clear that he taught no women, and the stories surrounding some of his legacy and how he handed it on have been little short of fantasy. His family have been constantly amazed and hurt by some of the claims that have been made, and it is interesting to note that the story has changed over the years.

Tom Bowen was undoubtedly a genius and I have an enormous respect for a man who stepped away from a steady income to follow his personal destiny, and faced criticism from some in his community as a result. He spent his life dedicated to helping others and never refused treatment to anyone who asked. He would be woken up in the middle of the night to help people, and invariably took no money for the treatments he performed.

His daughters, Pam Trigg and Heather Edmonds, have been a great source of encouragement and inspiration to me, and they have contributed much to the understanding of the man himself. Heather always said how amazed her father would be at the worldwide acceptance of a technique bearing his name. His humble approach and dedication to making the world a better place is an example to aspire to. A foundation helping disabled children continues to run in his name – the Tom Bowen legacy trust fund.

However, with a big deferential nod towards his memory, it is time to move on. We need to find a place for Bowen in the world, and need evidence and good scientific backup to do this. Anyone wishing to find out more about Tom Bowen the man can read Col Murray's well-researched book *In Search of Tom Bowen* (Murray 2010).

There is a fund in Tom Bowen's name, The Tom Bowen Legacy Trust Fund which exists to assist handicapped children, something close to Tom's heart.

For further details please contact:
TBLTF UK, Rosefield Clinic
1 Rosefield Mews, 42 Rosefield Street, Leamington Spa, CV32 4HE, U.K.

Email: info@TBLTF.org.uk   Tel: 01926 430 455

VARIATIONS ON A THEME

Over the years many variations of Bowen's work have popped up. Some of these have used the term 'Bowen'; others have renamed and rebranded themselves, using the success of others to promote their own versions. Whilst I think that any therapy that is effective and helpful has a place, it is somewhat galling to hear those who will put another therapy down in order to promote themselves.

"It is not Bowen – it is like Bowen but better." "It is an advanced version of Bowen." "Bowen's just the assessment – this is the treatment." I've heard all of these and many more from people who have come and gone, and made up lots of rubbish and lies along the way. An example of this is that Bowen's 'later work' has been claimed to be better than his earlier work, and therefore somehow 'advanced'. Illogical, and a little insulting to the man himself, quite apart from being unfounded.

Thousands of people around the world now lay claim to performing what they refer to as 'the Bowen Technique' or 'Bowen therapy'. It therefore strikes me as imperative that we establish some kind of common thread that runs through the practice carrying the name Bowen. As far as I'm concerned, if it doesn't carry the name Bowen, then it is not Bowen, however much people want to ride on the tails of it. It is therefore important for us to decide on something that we can all agree upon when we refer to the therapy, technique or method known as Bowen.

It strikes me that there are four key elements that make up and define Bowen: the distinct Bowen move itself, the stoppers or blockers, the breaks and the concept of not mixing the above with other methods. These will be defined in more detail in a later chapter, but the reason behind the statements is worth examining here. Most people who observed the man agree that some or all of these were elements he worked with. It seems that even with the more 'creative' interpretations of Bowen, all these are present in some degree.

These elements define a point from which we can now decide how far away we can stray while still having some kind of relationship with where we come from. It is a relationship that has been stretched to breaking point in some instances. To my thinking, if the hands-on approach contains a series of moves, includes breaks and stoppers, and discourages or does not permit other approaches to be mixed with these moves, then this is Bowen; if not, then even though there may be certain similarities, the relationship is not there.

ADVANCED BOWEN

Within the scope of the four elements that define Bowen, there is limitless potential for moves to be made in virtually any area of the body. Anyone who has undertaken a course of training at my college is given a series of procedures that serve as examples of what can be done. The examples are by no means exhaustive, and there is much more to be discovered.

A reasonably competent therapist with some body-reading skills and a good grasp of anatomy should be able to sensibly develop various treatment options, using the four Bowen elements as a guideline. Bowen himself would tell his trainees that what he was showing them was only a fraction of what there was. According to his daughter Heather, Bowen himself would come home and study anatomy books in order to work out where he was going wrong with a client. This suggests a work in progress, rather than a completed product.

It seems, however, that there are those who suggest that the teaching of more moves and more procedures by an experienced teacher enables these moves to somehow be defined as 'advanced Bowen'. Apart from being as impossible as, for instance, 'advanced air', this notion merely serves to exploit the gullible. There are some guidelines, of course, regarding how we go about changing the existing base work to tailor a treatment, and this is going to come from thoroughly knowing the groundwork and applying it consistently. But it doesn't offer a title. I have even found myself in the same room as people who themselves have been given the title Master of Bowen! This lofty title suggests a level of study, knowledge and application that I aspire to in my chosen therapy, but certainly not a title I would ascribe to myself.

Intrigued, I have probed these pinnacles of knowledge of the technique to which I have applied myself for over 20 years, in order to gain insights that have eluded me. Sadly what I find is people who, whilst no doubt willing and able therapists, have missed the irony of their title. When asked why one does something, the answer from people who have been teaching Bowen for some time is often: "Because Tom Bowen said so." It is not an answer that I, or any of my teachers, have ever given, and it insults the intelligence of the questioner.

If we can understand that simply adding more moves is somewhat naïve, how do we really advance? A common error of the beginner is to apply more procedures than are really needed. Chasing pain around the body, looking for the elusive magic bullet, the new Bowen therapist, more accustomed to spending lots of time and energy treating the client, goes on a rampage of procedures, adding more and more until the client can't take it any longer. This is often true of people who somehow feel guilty for not offering what they perceive as 'value for money'. More moves equates to better treatment, surely? Not always, and certainly not in the case of Bowen – an advanced student should be a reductionist.

Tom Bowen was famed for his ability to 'see' almost immediately where key imbalances lay. In treatments lasting only a few minutes he would apply small moves and then leave the room. Returning, he would then reassess, often sending the client home after only a mere handful of moves. Puzzled, the client often left the room in the same amount of pain as when they had arrived. Yet within the space of a few days, the pain would simply vanish and the problem would be resolved.

LOTS MORE MOVES BUT NOT ADVANCED ONES

This is the key to advancing. The advanced element does not come from the therapy in the form of more moves, but from the development of the therapist who must build his or her experience, sense of touch, listening and observation skills. Much of this can be taught, and examples can then be given of how to treat exactly what it is we see. More moves? Well, I have a stable of thousands of Bowen moves, none of which I found in a mystical drawer that I had forgotten about, but which have come about from working with clients and students, and from giving as examples when teaching. If the therapist can achieve what is needed with fewer moves, but better insight, then they are really getting to the root of what the man himself, Tom Bowen, was all about.

MIXING IT UP –
PRINCIPLES OF BOWEN AND COMMON GROUND

One of the most discussed, and in some cases controversial, aspects of Bowen is the argument as to whether or not Bowen mixes with other therapies. Furthermore, there is a certain point to which one can change Bowen around until it becomes something different. It is important to start with the understanding that the Bowen Technique is a therapy which has a worldwide following and acceptance, and is practised by many thousands of people. We therefore need, I feel, to define what it is that we call Bowen, and to at least determine that we are going to keep some kind of shape to that definition, if there is going to be a separate therapy called Bowen in ten years' time. The definition therefore has to come from what we see as the majority view. What is it that the majority of Bowen therapists are doing and how have these people been taught?

The nature of the argument has little or nothing to do with Tom Bowen. It might be that what we are doing bears little or no resemblance to what he was doing 30 years ago, and whilst that would be sad, it is not however my understanding. Even if it were, the therapy that thousands of people are now calling Bowen needs to be put into some kind of structure that can be identified, irrespective of what was being done a long time ago by one man.

We can call on what certain knowledge that we do have of Tom Bowen's modus operandi, coupled with the training content of the largest schools teaching Bowen around the world, and come up with something that most of us will recognise and relate to. More importantly will be Joe Public, who, when looking for a Bowen treatment, will be able to be relatively safe in the knowledge that what he has researched on the Internet as Bowen is what he is likely to receive when he turns up at the clinic advertising Bowen treatments. If I order a steak in a restaurant and get a plate of carrots I will be rightly aggrieved, even if the chef calls carrots 'steak' and thinks that carrots are better than steak. You can put a saddle on a pig but that doesn't make it a horse.

I have no doubt that there will be those who will disagree with the statements I am about to make in this regard, but take note that most of these people are those who have named their therapy something other than Bowen anyway, or call themselves advanced. In cycling terms it is called 'drafting': hanging on behind someone in front to ride their slipstream.

There are four elements which very clearly define Bowen:

1. The move – not a flick or a twang, but a rolling-type move designed to disturb the skin and underlying tissues. The move is a relatively light pressure, and no deep or prolonged pressure is used. If the move is consistently painful for the client, the therapist is applying Bowen incorrectly.

2. The stoppers – specific areas which use the potential energy of structure, discussed in detail elsewhere in this book.

3. The breaks – short pauses designed to allow the appropriate response to take place within the body. The key element of Bowen, the breaks should be at least two to three minutes long.

4. No other hands-on treatments – a point that Tom Bowen was very specific about. "Don't see anyone else" is the advice given, and a theory that has been tested to death over the years by many therapists and clients.

These four elements clearly define what Bowen is and therefore what Bowen is not. Far from being a restrictive and controlling edict, it is in fact very liberating, as much by what it doesn't say as what it does.

The first three of these areas are covered in other sections of this book, but it is number four that seems to provoke the most controversy and resistance amongst the mixers out there. The therapists, and I have met hundreds of them, who tell me that they do 'Bowen' but do it 'differently' or 'better', are generally the ones who have learned several therapies and see good results with most or all of them. The next step, therefore, is to create a blend of these treatments that yield great results and keep the client happy and the therapist busy and feeling that they are giving good value. I can honestly say that I have absolutely no problem with this. A bit of reflexology, some massage, a few Bowen moves here and a chiropractic adjustment there. If this works, bring it on and pay the choir.

My simple point, however, is that it is not Bowen. It does not fall within the remit of Bowen, it is not recognisable as what thousands of people all over the world call Bowen and it would not be what a client who had researched the technique would be expecting when they booked a treatment. I would never for a moment suggest that someone cannot or should not mix Bowen with whatever they please, but simply that, when they do so, they should respect the therapy, the other people using the therapy and the client who is paying for the treatment, by being clear about what it is that they are really doing. Otherwise, it is both misleading and a little dishonest.

Bowen mixed with any other physical therapy, however effective, useful or inspired, is just not Bowen. The mixture doesn't make the treatment any less valid; it simply steps away from the definition of what is very widely accepted as the Bowen Technique. That said, there are many theories, applications and approaches that encompass the understanding of the technique, and create an ability to be incredibly varied and creative in one's application. For instance, I might have studied acupuncture, kinesiology and Bowen. I muscle test for an imbalance in a meridian, then find a specific acupuncture point and apply a Bowen move in the area to release this. Am I mixing and stepping outside the definition of Bowen? Well, if we check the rules, I have applied a move after the stoppers, put a break in and not done any other physical therapy, so the answer is no – it is still Bowen, just with some diagnostic and assessment elements included.

CHANGING THE RULES

For many therapists the learning of Bowen follows a fairly rigid formula: there are certain procedures, with specific moves in very clearly defined sequences. They are told that this is the only way to apply the procedures and that they will eventually be taught 'advanced' moves which follow on from the original rigid secrets. In addition, they are told that if they stray from this designated pathway, they are 'doing it wrong' – fear is a great tool of control! This is not the case of course. Tom Bowen did not stick rigidly to a series of procedures, but approached the work from the perspective of working out where a problem or imbalance lay, releasing it and letting the body sort out where to make changes. He constantly picked up and put down ideas, and it is likely that his work today would be radically different from that of 50 years ago.

A training course does, however, need structure, and this structure can then be tested and duplicated to create a standard within the field and a recognisable way of working. But the procedures which all students are initially taught are little more than very good examples of how the whole principle of soft tissue release hangs together. One of my most important sayings is: "Bowen is a system of bodywork, not a series of procedures!" This helps to sum up the big difference between myself and other Bowen teachers – and it is a big difference. If I stuck to the original procedures, with perhaps a dozen more thrown in for good measure as part of a mythical 'advanced' course, then within a very short space of time I would run out of ideas for treatment and be bored rigid by the parameters imposed on me. Some people already experience this.

Instead, I teach students that we need to develop ourselves as bodyworkers first and foremost:

• Learn to look at the body to see where movements happen, where limitations exist and where they come from.

• Feel for changes in the tissues.

• Observe shifts in muscle and connective tissue contractions and movement patterns.

• Work creatively as the body changes.

If we can develop these skills, then the moves that we make, whatever the therapy, will probably be effective. There are simply no advanced moves in Bowen – it is a contradiction in terms. Nevertheless, there are advanced therapists, and anyone can take on this advancement and never even need to learn another procedure.

There are certain guidelines and rules, however, that one needs to follow in order to be able to mix and match the procedures, and the first call is to learn the basics thoroughly. The beauty of Bowen is that, even at the beginning stages, students will get superb results very quickly. Whilst this is gratifying, the later stage of being able to get the same results with half the work is even more exciting. It is developing intuitive and creative bodyworkers rather than training monkeys that interests me.

Each procedure is made up of individual moves, and each move has a function, a response and a reason for being there. It has been a long journey for me in trying to discover the reason for the profound effects that happen when I use such a light touch and do so little hands-on work. Over the years I have been exposed to hundreds of different approaches to doing bodywork, yet have found no reason to move outside the field that I call Bowen to seek more therapies, or to add hundreds more procedures to a repertoire. If anything, I think Bowen is the single most profound and simple method for changing tissues and body structures. My mission has been to develop and explain the reasons why we do what we do, and perhaps why they work; this book is part of the journey. Ultimately, my mission is to help people to see how to get there by themselves and surpass their teacher. Give a man a fish.

CHAPTER 4

The Bowen Move

The Bowen move is what defines the technique and is made up of three parts:

1. The skin slack

2. The pressure

3. The rolling-type move

THE SKIN SLACK

The skin slack is what we use in order to carry out the move itself, and in this respect it works for us. However, the spare skin covering the tissue that we are trying to move can also work against us as well, as it can create a barrier to the completion of the move. To get at the muscle, we need to pull (or push) the skin in the opposite direction to the move, before effectively 'riding' it over the tendon, ligament or muscle which is the target of our move. When we make the move we must ensure that we don't slide over the surface of the skin. If we think of our fingers as being glued to the skin, we can imagine that, when we get to the limit of the skin, we are stopped, before any sliding can occur.

The pressure needed to move the skin around is very slight – much less than the pressure used to make the move. The other factor to remember about skin slack is the variability factor of skin availability. In addition, the tissues that are adhered to the underside of the skin, referred to as superficial fascia or the adipose layer, will vary greatly in thickness and texture. Whenever we move the skin, we also move this underlying tissue as well. In some people, and in certain areas of the body, there will be lots of skin available to move around – possibly even too much! The average amount will be similar to that available on the back of the hand, and yet, with some clients, the amount will be more like that found on the palm. This variability will inevitably affect the quality and content of the move, but it is important that the pressure is not increased simply because of a lack of skin slack.

Skin slack also has implications for observation, as the skin is the largest organ of the body and is the end point for all the other organs of the body. In the case of the kidneys, the skin is the regulation co-ordinator for temperature and general conditions outside. It responds to the autonomic nervous system (ANS) and can be measured to test the function and effectiveness of a huge number of systems of the body. Furthermore, it is intimately connected to a major endocrine organ – the adipose layer, or superficial fascia.

We can make good use of observations regarding the condition of the skin and its temperature, colour and elasticity. Does it have blemishes or textures that are noticeable? When we have made the moves, the first response to them is often indicated by the skin. Redness, or erythema, which develops from the capillaries in the deeper layers of the skin, can be a sign that significant changes are taking place and that a response might be required. The skin is a constantly changing structure that begs close observation during treatment and which, if we are paying attention, will give us great rewards.

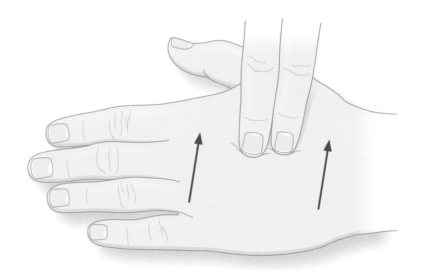

Here the skin slack is drawn in the opposite direction to the intended move. Only at the point of the move will the 'eyeball pressure' be applied.

THE PRESSURE

The variable pressures used in Bowen have been the subject of much discussion and debate. The idea about what Tom Bowen did or did not do has had to give way to the weight of clinical application from thousands of Bowen therapists all over the world.

These days, Bowen is described and widely accepted as a 'light touch therapy'. Whilst there has been much disagreement over the years as to what constitutes light touch, I am going to go out on a limb and say that, for the sake of argument, 'touch' refers to the physical touch of the client by the therapist. At the same time, I recognise and freely defer to the energetic field of the human form, and accept that the influence of the therapist stems from more than just a physical touch. So please, no letters!

The pressure used when making a Bowen move is one which could best be described as confident, without being hard. The phrase 'eyeball pressure' is sometimes used to describe this pressure, yet if you were to press onto your eye and then feel the average Bowen move, you would find that generally there is much more pressure used in the latter than what could be safely applied to an eye. Nonetheless the term is a useful one, as it can be used to describe a type of pressure. If you press your eyeball then it will become quickly apparent that any excessive pressure will be painful and damaging. But, as you are pressing, you will notice that there is a point at which the pressure is acceptable. The action of finger pressing and the eye being pressed communicate that a comfortable level has been reached and that the pressing should now stop. At this level the finger could probably be easily moved around on the skin covering the eye without discomfort.

We can also see that there is much less pressure needed for us to simply take the skin slack, and so it emerges that there are two types of pressure required when making a Bowen move: one type to take the skin slack and the other to make the move. It might sound obvious, but it is a difference that is easily missed. An experienced therapist will constantly be aware of the pressure differentiation and be sure not to apply such pressure as to accidentally flick a muscle while taking the skin slack.

The pressure used will naturally vary from person to person and from body type to body type. A rugby player's hamstrings would probably need the application of more pressure than a ballerina's. That said, if the rugby player was injured and in a lot of pain, I would need to reduce the level of pressure so as not to hurt him. Indeed, I might even back off to the extent that it would be a feather-light touch. Bowen is ideal for use specifically in very acute conditions because very little pressure is required for the move to be effective, and for the repair process to begin. If in doubt about the amount of pressure needed, then follow the principle that applies to virtually everything in Bowen: less is more.

As well as the actual pressure applied by the fingers or thumbs, heaviness in a move can also come from tension in the hands, arms or shoulders; it is therefore important to ensure that these areas are relaxed when performing the moves. Tension will translate into the hands very easily, resulting in a heavy or hard move.

The concept of pressure becomes increasingly important as we begin to understand the layers of the skin and superficial fascia and their role in a whole-body treatment. The superficial fascia, or adipose layer, acts as a protection for the deeper layers, and this aspect needs to be acknowledged by the therapist if the deeper structures are to be accessed. Pressing too hard and too fast results in this fluffy layer acting as a crash mat, stopping the progression of the force into the body. Some forms of bodywork, and even some 'developed' or 'later' forms of Bowen, mistakenly apply much more pressure than necessary or even useful. The result is likely to be painful and potentially damaging, especially in the hands of unskilled and thoughtless practitioners.

It is surprising how deep you can go if you are patient, acknowledge each layer and effectively 'ask permission' before going any deeper, stopping and working wherever you happen to be if permission is not granted. It is this intelligence of touch that determines an advanced practitioner, rather than the number of procedures learned or workshops attended. Whilst Bowen is described as a light touch, it would be a mistake to assume that depth is not possible. Thinking and listening through our fingers is what is called for in order to detect changes and tensions in the layers we are working through.

THE ROLLING-TYPE MOVE

The idea of the actual move is to create a muscle disturbance on which the brain will probably need to take action. This disturbance creates questions that need answers, and this questioning and responding happens during the breaks in treatment. The actual response and the way that information is shared throughout the various systems, particularly the influence of deep fascia, is under some consideration right now. A new understanding of this deep layer has given rise to suggestions that perhaps it is the deeper fascia which is responsible for much of the muscular communication to and from the brain. Certainly, this material is there for a reason. However, given the lack of definitive research at this time, we will stay with the muscle–brain model. Check back in a few years!

The quality of the move is determined by two elements: speed and pressure. If the move is performed too fast and with too much pressure, the result will be a flick or a twang. Try it on yourself and see the difference. If we flick the muscle, the chances of causing pain are very high, and the body will take action appropriate to the circumstances. Instead of creating a space for asking questions to determine an action, the response will be one that closes or defends against the pain, and the aim of the Bowen move will not be achieved.

Again, we must remember that the move should only be made within the limits of the skin available, and sliding must not happen during the move. Defining 'sliding' is quite easy: if your thumbs or fingers travel from the point of application, and end in a different place, then you have made a sliding move. The fingers need to be fixed at all times, as if stuck to the surface of the skin.

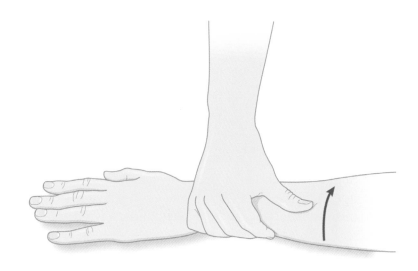

Skin slack preceding the rolling-type move.

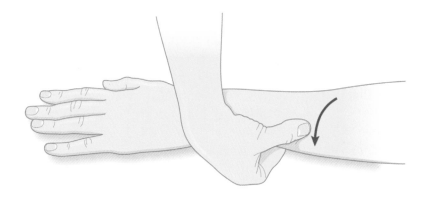

End of the rolling-type move.

The rolling-type move, although gentle, is still very dynamic. It is not really enough for the thumbs to push over the underlying tissue – the hands need to move as well. The whole of the surface of the thumb or finger makes the move and controls it at the same time. The action of the move creates an equal and opposite reaction in the muscle. Consequently, as we move (for instance) medially, the muscle that has been challenged rolls laterally, away from the pressure and direction of the move.

Ideally, the move should be made on the exhalation of the client (and possibly the therapist if there is tension present); it should take around two full seconds to perform, from the beginning of the move to the end. When the move is completed, a slight pause is recommended before either going on to the next move or moving away from the body, giving the therapist a moment to take in what has just happened and, if necessary, to stop. The move is a little like a swing in tennis or golf: once the actual hitting has been accomplished, the emphasis is on timing the stroke for maximum effect. The Bowen move is an art form in itself, and a good move is a pleasure to receive and to perform.

There will always be significant variation in the quality of the move, with the feeling changing from person to person and from one part of the body to another. In the case of a client who has a lot of adipose tissue in a certain area, the muscle that we are trying to disturb will naturally be well covered, and it won't always be possible to feel much, if anything at all. In this instance it is important not to try to apply a greater pressure to perform the move, but to work within the confines of what is available, keeping to the gentle pressure and trying to carry out a move which will create some degree of disturbance. It can admittedly be very frustrating, but the approach is nevertheless still highly effective, as the body still needs to investigate what is going on within it. Patience is required here. The superficial fluffy tissues will give way if gently persuaded, but will close up like a clam at high tide if you push on them too hard. The key to accomplishing an effective move is practice. It may look very simple, but achieving the perfect move can take a long time, and timing is crucial.

DIRECTION OF THE MOVE

A question often asked is whether the direction of the move being made makes a difference. With the exception of the moves in Page Two along the erector spinae (see p.55), I would have to say probably not. The direction of most of the moves is determined by it simply being the easiest way to go, or where it is possible to move. For instance, the move over the ITB in Page One (see p.48) is written as being a posterior move. However, if I were treating a client in a chair, it would be ridiculous to attempt to make a posterior move. Anatomically it makes no sense either, as the ITB is simply a created sculpture anyway, and moving in one direction or another is really not going to make any difference. But in the case of the last diaphragm move (see p.87), there is only one direction to go, and so the logic of direction comes into play.

Similarly, the order of some moves is little short of arbitrary, and it makes very little difference whether the first move on a knee is performed medially or laterally. However, as a note to those just starting to learn Bowen, there are points at which it is important to work in a certain sequence and direction, so it is preferable to learn the work in the order taught, before deciding to meddle too much with the sequences.

It is said that Bowen moves are generally 'cross fibre' in direction. If we are going to refer solely to muscles, it is true that a Bowen move is rarely in the direction of muscular contraction. However, the nature of fascia is that it covers muscular structures and travels in every conceivable direction. Hence it is somewhat tricky to limit the movement to a direction that is perpendicular to a given muscle. The Bowen Technique is a difficult creature to pin down, and when one starts to look for consistencies in order to find some definition, it goes off on a tangent, and starts to provide exceptions to any rule directed at it.

SIZE MATTERS

In this day and age it is quite likely that we are going to come across clients who are, if not obese, then at least quite large. Carrying substantial amounts of adipose tissue, these clients present challenges in terms of how much pressure we should apply. The analogy I propose is that of trying to make a move on the palm of the hand. There is little or no movement, and the whole process is frustrating and unsatisfactory. Yet the alternative, to apply lots of pressure to try to 'get in' and feel underlying tissues, is counterproductive. Similarly, applying heavier pressure to these types of client is more likely to make them feel unwell, achy and nauseous.

Whilst I acknowledge that a treatment using light pressure may feel less than satisfactory, it is important that the temptation to apply more pressure and go deeper is resisted. I have discussed the implications of deep pressure in the section relating to superficial fascia (see p.35), but it's a point worth repeating here. A light touch does not exclude depth. By gently dropping through and acknowledging the layers of the body as we go down, we create an explicit permission. At each stage we are asking the body if it is okay to keep going, thereby establishing co-operation and unity.

Bowen is regarded as a light touch therapy, and indeed it is. I would therefore challenge any therapist who considers themselves to have better access to the body because they are a 'deep tissue' therapist to think again. Simply put, pressing hard does not get you in further. In fact the opposite is more accurate: the harder you press, the more you stay on the surface, mainly thanks to the incredible resilience of the adipose, or superficial, layer. This light fluffy layer doesn't seem like much, yet it has the ability to both store and absorb energy in the form of pressure. If you slip over on the ice and land on your behind, you can thank the superficial fascia for your pelvis not being smashed. If the adipose layer can withstand being subjected to the pressure of many kilograms, it will be child's play for it to oppose a heavy-handed therapist trying to grind their way through.

THE BREAKS

There are two types of break in Bowen that we need to address. Firstly, there is the break that is most noticeable – the therapist leaving the room in between sets of moves, for which Bowen is famed. It has been suggested, somewhat cynically in my opinion, that Tom Bowen only did this in order to be able to treat from two or three rooms. Whilst the ability to conduct multiple treatments is a bonus stemming from the breaks, it is by no means the only one. Several theories have been put forward to explain the reason for the breaks, and this book seems the ideal forum in which to explore these.

The second break represents the amount of time necessary between treatments, ideally a week but no longer than ten days. Research has shown that the effects of Bowen continue over a period of a week. A constant bombardment of the nervous systems of the body with information might impair the process of self-adjustment that seems to be an integral part of Bowen.

BREAKS BETWEEN SETS OF MOVES

In the discussion of traditional anatomy in Chapter 2, we mentioned the Galenic belief, still held today, that structural movement is mediated by the brain. There are therefore many leaps that we make alongside this belief, one of them being that if sensation is a function of central nervous system and cranial function, then this must also be true of all things related to sensation. So the idea of the breaks is that we are in some way communicating with the brain on a more subconscious level. The breaks give the body the time to communicate with the brain using what I have termed the 'ARM' – the appropriate response mechanism.

We actually rely on ARMs on a moment-to-moment basis throughout the day, and use them to feel and appear normal. If you are walking down the street and someone in a car toots their horn at you and waves, your immediate (and appropriate) response is to wave back, maybe even smiling. You may even do this without having a clue as to who the person was in the car, such is the conditioned response. Imagine you are at an event or a function, and someone walks up to you with his or her hand outstretched; you shake it – an appropriate response. If, however, I walked up to you without ever having met you before, my arms open for a big hug, your appropriate response would probably be to avoid that hug at all costs and protect yourself – an appropriate response to an inappropriate action.

We do this kind of judging all the time, questioning the information that arrives at the brain and working out how it should be responded to. The older we get and the more experience we have, the more these situations are easily recognisable and dealt with. When we were four, we may well have hugged the other four-year-old we didn't know, simply because we hugged everyone. As we get older, this approach sadly has its drawbacks and we learn to moderate our behaviour. Over time we build up a memory bank of what is appropriate and when, and we modify the stored information as necessary. Slowly the hot-headed youth, impatient for change, learns to adapt what they consider to be appropriate.

Something similar happens in a Bowen situation. A series of moves are followed by a break, during which the practitioner leaves the room. This break should be in the region of two minutes as a minimum, but longer in some situations. It is this break which seems to actually create the effectiveness of the work and allow such a limited amount of work to be effective. Once the hands are off the body and the therapist out of the room, the brain and body can begin a dialogue.

Brain: What was that?

Body: Not sure, never experienced anything like that.

Brain: Okay, let's check this out. Was it a stroke sort of feeling?

Body: No.

Brain: A massage?

Body: Definitely not.

Brain: Did it tickle?

Body: Of course not, I'd have told you if it did.

Brain: OK, don't snap. Did it hurt?

Body: No, not really … not at all in fact.

Brain: Right answer. So, err … was it erotic?

Body: No! So embarrassing.

Brain: OK, I'm stuck here as to how to respond.

Body: Well, do you have to respond at all?

Brain: Are you mad? Of course I have to respond. Something has happened. Someone put their hands on you and has done something. I can hardly let that go now can I?

Body: S'pose not.

Brain: Right, you stay there. I'll send out some other signals, and find out what's related and what else has been done, and then get back to you. I'll whack down some nerve-ending blood while we're waiting, just to see if anything more informative comes back. You are very trying … did you know that?

Body: Okay, sorreee … Jeez!

Well that's how it happens in my mind. Clients then tend to fall asleep, which isn't really sleep or deep sleep, but is a shutting down of the primary motor cortex in order for other information to be exchanged. Common responses will be an increase in blood to the skin, or erythema, but also, interestingly enough, other untreated areas can also 'pink up'. Invariably the client will start to relax deeply and may well fall into what appears to be quite a sound sleep.

In fact this is more likely to be a parasympathetic nervous system response with the client able to respond readily if needs be. It takes some time to drop into deep sleep with the body carrying out a series of checks to ensure that it is safe to do so. Am I warm enough or safe enough? Am I hungry or do I need to go to the toilet? It is like when we fall asleep on the train: although the sleep is there, we can readily respond when it is time to get off the train, or if someone talks to us.

Short periods of this napping type of sleep are very refreshing and creative, and the 'power nap' as it has become known is one of the better things you can do for yourself during the day (Hayashi, Motoyoshi and Hori 2005). This sleep is also more likely if the therapist leaves the room, allowing the system to really take stock and work out what has just happened when the tissues were disturbed by the rolling-type Bowen move.

I therefore find that two things are beneficial: firstly, the break immediately after the first moves is slightly longer than the prescribed two minutes; and, secondly, I ensure that the client has their eyes loosely closed. It is very hard for the body to move towards a parasympathetic state if the eyes are open. There is a good reason why meditation is done with the eyes closed or mostly closed. The client who sits up on their arms, eyes open and looking around the room, is likely to have less of a response than the more relaxed one. A lot of this is about conditions and the right environment in which to treat, but I would suggest that, even in the most chaotic situations, a client with their eyes closed has a very good chance of dropping off when the first moves are applied.

As well as initiating the brain–body dialogue, the breaks have an effect on the tension of the connective tissue, in particular the fascia. Fascia is made up of a triple helix-type structure, wound into tension and held all over the body – a spiral, crossing over and under other spiralling structures. The more tension that is present, either through injury or other stressors, emotional included, the more energy is present in these tightly wound, spring-like structures. Like a jack-in-the-box, little pressure or movement is required to release this energy, but, in the case of the spiral fascia, the release is generally a little less dramatic, although this is not always so. The unwinding of this fascia can happen very slowly, over a period of days or even weeks; or it can happen as the client lies on the couch, with cases of spontaneous twisting and involuntary movement of limbs having been recorded.

Research into the effects of the Bowen Technique on hamstring flexibility has shown an immediate increase in flexibility straight after the treatment (Marr et al. 2011). Not only was this change in flexibility maintained in all the treated cases, but also, in some instances, the increase continued over seven days. This is a unique result for a passive treatment, and suggests that the continuing change is prompted by the Bowen move. Another good reason to leave well alone and not mix in other therapies during the break between Bowen treatments.

When we first begin learning Bowen, the breaks are given and written down as to where they are taken and for how long. However, as we start to progress, and develop an intuitive feel for the people we are working on, we can start to put breaks in the treatment wherever it feels right. If you find yourself asking the question "What shall I do next?", then the answer is probably "Do nothing, get your hands off and get out of the room". Learning to take your hands off and put in a break when you find yourself overworking is probably one of the greatest skills you can learn; in my opinion this defines you as an advanced Bowen therapist much more than any extra moves you might have learned on a course.

TIME BETWEEN TREATMENTS

Five to ten days seems to be the optimum time between treatments. In some instances, however, clients will benefit from breaks of three weeks, and often change dramatically in that time without even noticing the changes! I am often telling students that the most common response from a client will be: "Well I don't think it is anything to do with what you did, but I do feel so much better." The insignificance of what little work the therapist did compared to the degree of change experienced by the client just don't add up. In many cases the client will have forgotten what the original problem was or the severity of it. This is a good reason to take structured notes and records, something we will deal with in due course (see Chapter 21).

It is generally accepted by those who have been practising Bowen for any length of time that the client and therapist will see some degree of change within the space of, on average, three or four treatments. This, however, is a claim that needs to be qualified and built on. And whilst it is not unusual in acute situations to find that there is a rapid response to treatment, there are certain circumstances where an extended course of treatment will be needed.

If a client presents with back pains that have troubled them for many years, it is fairly evident that a change in their functional behaviour has taken place. Whilst Bowen is going to be a very effective tool in treating pain levels, we need to bear in mind that other factors – such as changes in muscle tone, strength and the ability to move normally – must be addressed. It is possible that other professionals might need to be consulted if the individual Bowen therapist does not have the required skills in these departments. I have always maintained that skilled referral – the ability for any individual to realise and accept their own limitations, and to find and surround themselves with those that are qualified and equipped – is a skill as well as a demonstration of humility.

Patience is a required skill when looking for changes. Pain is only one indicator and we need to be skilful in our observations and our ability to read the body. Once again, effective and detailed note-taking is required, as often the only way we can demonstrate change is to refer to notes taken in previous sessions.

Asking clients to return for treatment is also something that is potentially of great benefit. A client who has had relief from aches and pains can hardly be expected to stay the same for weeks and weeks, once their normal routine has been resumed. I therefore advise clients to return every six to eight weeks for top-up treatments, which help them to not only maintain their improvements, but also prevent the return of any injuries. This is particularly useful when dealing with sports people, who are prone to injury and loss of training time. I firmly believe that Bowen is a particularly effective treatment for long-term sports injury prevention. Athletes being treated with Bowen report remarkable responses in terms of fewer injuries, as well as faster recovery after any minor injuries.

Other areas in which more frequent treatment might be indicated or useful is palliative care. The main concern here is to keep the client comfortable while attempting to manage pain and reduce reliance on medication where possible. Pregnancy is another situation where more frequent treatment is possible and also very useful. A woman experiencing back pain, particularly in the final trimester of pregnancy, can return to treatments on, say, a daily basis if need be.

BEWARE THE LIST

Something I have shied away from over the years, and to this day still do, is the making of lists of procedures to address certain problems. I accept that this approach might at some stage seem useful, but to my mind it completely misses the point of what we are trying to achieve. The law of natural cure states that the body be treated as a whole without referral to named diseases. Whilst specific issues or problems might be a starting point from which to investigate, no two people are going to be the same.

A list of procedures for specific problems creates the same reductionist approach which has plagued medicine since time immemorial. It is the reason why we have people with back pain, who get treated over and over again for this particular complaint and nothing else. Logic should tell us to back away and find out what else is going on, but the blinkered idea that pain comes from the place that it is being experienced limits this thinking. Why then would we want to approach a holistic system of treatment from the same skewed perspective?

The four rules of all complementary therapy should be:

1. We do not diagnose.

2. We do not treat specific conditions.

3. We do not alter or prescribe medications unless qualified to do so.

4. We do not make claims regarding the benefit, efficacy or outcomes of our treatment unless there is scientific evidence to back them up.

A person presenting with whiplash will have a whole history of other issues and a life that has brought them to this point. It might be that we will use a reasonably standard set of approaches, but it is easy to miss things. Someone recently told me of a client they had treated with an ankle procedure. The weekly migraines that the client had suffered for over 15 years vanished. Could this be explained anatomically? Absolutely, although I'm not going to try to do so here. Does this mean that an ankle procedure is something that we should do for migraines? Possibly.

A list is a dangerous thing when it comes to treating people rather than conditions, and should be avoided wherever possible. There is a temptation to use the list and become prescriptive. Instead, start to think outside the box and look for what's not obvious, especially when things aren't changing the way you would expect them to.

Pages One, Two and Three will be covered in the next three chapters: they form the foundation of the Bowen method of bodywork and need to be fully mastered. They are nearly always performed as the first treatment, and are generally prerequisites for the other procedures.

CHAPTER 5

Page One

There isn't really a better name for this procedure than Page One. As with the first page of a novel it sets the scene and grabs the interest of the reader. At the same time, the lack of a particular name or body region means that the possibilities are not limited in terms of where the effects might be seen. In some schools the term BRM, or basic relaxation move, has been used for Pages One to Three. This rather misses the power and profound nature of these pages, and reduces them to simple and basic work, to be got out of the way before the important stuff. It is a little like saying that Mozart was a musician who wrote some nice tunes.

Page One has several moves which are key to the success of the whole treatment, and need to be studied and practised at length if we are to understand why this work is so important. It is the first entry onto the body and has several purposes. The first aim is to work on the stress-loading areas of the lower back in order to access some of the stored energy in this area. These first moves, which serve to introduce the therapist to the client and vice versa, are probably the most important and profound in the entire repertoire of Bowen moves. These moves are commonly referred to as stoppers or blockers.

THE STOPPERS

Humans are the only mammals that stand upright, demonstrating our superiority over the rest of the animal kingdom. We expose all the areas of vulnerability that, if we had any natural predators, we would need to keep protected from attack. This evolutionary success, however, comes at a price, as we consequently have to maintain a curved spine in order to absorb the pressures that gravity places upon it. The curves of the spine act as shock absorbers and allow us to run, walk, jump and generally bounce around.

As with any shock absorber, there will be more stress loading on some areas than others; in the case of the human spine, these are the apexes of the spinal curves. In these areas the stress loading is at its greatest, and the tissues supporting and surrounding these points will be highly energetic. A feature of virtually all the moves of Pages One, Two and Three is that they are made on highly stress-loaded areas of the body. These are areas where there is often tension and tenderness – typical indications of loading. The stoppers are specifically made around the apexes of the spinal curves in order to take advantage of this stress loading on the spine.

The term 'stoppers' is a bit of a misnomer, because they neither stop nor block, as was at one time suggested. If anything, they open, since they move over the erector spinae, where the thoracolumbar fascia (TLF) blends in with the rest of the spinal and abdominal muscles and fascia. Even tissues from the hamstrings and lower dorsal sacroiliac (SI) ligament can be found in this area, and they make up a major part of the tensional components.

After performing stopper moves, their effects can nearly always be seen and felt within a very short time. Redness, or erythema, in the area is often evident, but even in the absence of this, an increase in heat can usually be felt. This can be seen as an energetic change or release, and an indicator that change is afoot. I am generally reluctant within the field of complementary and alternative therapies (CAMs) to use the word 'energy', as it is a widely abused term that has some dubious uses attached to it. For this discussion we need to stick firmly to Newtonian laws and not get into the esoteric ideas of energy or its movement. I should also say that I do embrace much of the idea that Newtonian physics is as reductionist in its approach as a standardised study of anatomy. However, for the purpose of this book, I intend to avoid quantum physics and esoteric leaps, which, whilst fascinating, are way beyond my simple brain, and I leave it to people like James Oschman to explain it better than I ever could (Oschman 2000).

When we talk about energy, we need to remember some simple rules regarding this entity and what you can or can't do with it. Firstly, energy cannot be created and therefore cannot be destroyed. What we can do is convert or divert it, and the stoppers are located in such places as to give easy access to a huge store of structural energy. Secondly, energy in the body, and anywhere else for that matter, is either potential (stored) energy or kinetic (moving) energy. In this instance, energy that has been applied to tissues of the body is in the process of translation or conversion.

The area of the first stoppers, below the second lumbar vertebra, is referred to in Chinese Medicine as *Ming Men*: 'Gate of the Fire of Life' or 'Gate of Vitality'. It refers to a passageway representing a place where *qi* or energy can enter and exit, hence the reference to gates. It is also referred to as the meeting point of fire and water – steam being the powerful product of such a meeting. When we make the gentle rolling-type moves over this area, we release and open its energetic potential and allow it to be a focus point for the rest of the lower body. From a structural perspective, the stoppers are also very important as remedial moves in their own right. We often come across significant tightness or spasm in the lower back, and most non-specific lower-back pain presentations will involve this area.

Lower limb presentations will also often have an origin or involvement in the lower back or sacrum, and the stoppers are a starting point for understanding that this fuse box-type arrangement is vitally important for body-wide functional balance. The implications for the whole body are therefore tremendous. If the tightest or most stressed point of the spine is relaxed, there is an immediate knock-on effect for the whole of the spinous process. Given that the nerves of function for the entire system stem from the spine, any relaxation in associated spinal muscles creates the possibility that there will be a change to the entire system, simply by the application of two moves.

The effect of the stopper is such that it is highly unlikely that a treatment would be given which didn't include the lower stoppers as the first moves. That said, the lower stoppers are always performed before the upper ones. Although we could happily perform the upper stoppers without the lower ones, if we are to see the full energetic effect, we need to open up the energy storehouse lower down first.

It is important to understand the areas that we are treating. Page One is a starting point in another way, as it is a prerequisite for a lot of other procedures, such as the knee, hamstring, pelvis and sacrum. However, even without these additional procedures, clients presenting with lower-back pain, knee presentations, ankle imbalances and pelvic distortions can all potentially respond with Page One. Pages One to Three form a complete body treatment, taking into account most of the stress-loading areas of the system; they should form the basis for a first treatment, with only a few more, if any, procedures needed.

The first two moves (moves 1 and 2) of Page One – the lower and upper stoppers – should be considered to be the first two moves of every treatment performed, irrespective of presentation. Moves 3 and 4 are slightly different from the norm: for these, the area we work on is where all the gluteal muscles conjoin. This is an area that is covered with quite a lot of adipose tissue and superficial fascia, with the actual muscle being quite deep, even in slim people. If we try to roll over the grouping as in an ordinary move, then the pressure is released and we will not feel the little lump signifying that we are in the right location.

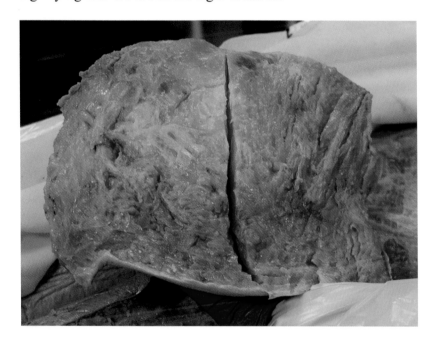

Just how much superficial fascia covers the gluteal area is shown here. The depth of this tissue is nearly 6 cm and has no muscle in it. The surface of the gluteus maximus can be seen at the right edge of the picture.

The correct move is instead more of a push, allowing us to almost jump over this grouping. It should be quite clear and defined. Caution should be exercised in order not to come too far to the side of the body and work over the hip area by mistake. As these structures can feel similar, it is an easy mistake to make, but practising palpation around the hip joint should eventually clarify the difference. An excellent reference book for this area is *The Trail Guide to the Body* by Andrew Biel (2005).

While performing these moves it is important to try to create some form of assessment of what it is that you are feeling. How does one side compare to the other? Is there any difference in temperature, muscle tone, tissue tension and so forth? This kind of information is not gathered from a judgemental or diagnostic perspective, but simply for creating a continuous comparison from one move to another, and from one treatment session to the next. The gluteal moves will often change quite dramatically during the treatment, and this should be noted as and when it occurs.

Moves 5 and 6 are the back of the knee and the ITB. The move at the back of the knee is performed level with the top of the patella, or kneecap, and not at the bend of the leg. A reading will be triggered at the holding point on the ischial tuberosity. This reading can often be tricky to pick up, but moving the holding hand slightly medially will put your hands into a small bridging area between the biceps femoris and the sacrotuberous (ST) ligament. It is here that you will get the reading, but only if you are concentrating into the holding-point hand. The head of the biceps femoris is in fact continuous with the ST ligament, and the implications of this will be pointed out in the discussion of the hamstrings in Chapter 13.

It can be quite tricky to feel the reading at the conjoined tendon of the biceps femoris and semitendinosus, as it is very subtle. However, this will come with practice and concentration, but the main secret is not to hold too hard or to flick the biceps femoris tendon at the knee. The move at the back of the knee releases the strong storage container of energy in the stress-loaded area of the popliteal fossa. This is then made available to the rest of the leg and utilised when the last move is made.

The last move is over the structure referred to as the iliotibial band, or ITB. In most anatomical charts this band can be seen as a distinct structure, rising from the knee and attaching to the gluteal region posteriorly and to the quadriceps at the front. In reality, the ITB is part of a continuous fascial stocking which wraps itself around the leg and has tensional fibres running perpendicular to it, through the fabric of the tissue. Thus, as an independent structure, the ITB does not exist in the way that it is portrayed, which is good news for Bowen therapists, since we are able to determine the point at which the move is most likely to have its greatest effect and accordingly be successful. The margin for error is therefore less than for most of the other moves; the move can even be located in other areas to use the energy released by the first move across the popliteal fossa.

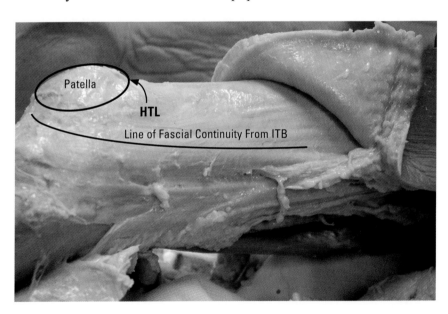

Fascial continuity of the ITB where it blends around the knee as a continuous band.

The 'hit the lat' (HTL) move is performed when the client is turned over and effectively completes Page One. Here 'lat' refers to the lateral inferior border of the vastus lateralis, which is also the conjoined tendon of the quadriceps femoris. Again, from a traditional anatomical perspective, this is clearly defined on a muscle chart and can be tracked. From a more realistic, fascial point of view, the lat is part of the fascia lata stocking, and is under a lot of physical and structural strain around the edge of the patella. The fascia at this point, however, joins up with the fascial bags of all the muscles of the leg and groin, and potentially creates a clear relationship with the pelvic floor and abdomen. It might explain why we so often hear the stomach gurgle when the HTL move is performed.

It is interesting to look at the HTL in terms of how it links in with areas such as the ankle, particularly when considered with the complete nature of the tissue surrounding the leg. The kneecap is encased in strong binding fascia, which creates multiple directions of strain and movement. The muscle at this point is very small and ill-defined, and the feeling we have of rolling over it is much more to do with the connective structures surrounding it than with any muscle.

The lat forms the first move of several other procedures, mainly owing to its big energy storage but also because it links the lower and upper legs effectively. It can also serve as a treatment for the knee as a stand-alone. On many occasions I have 'hit the lat' on someone's painful knee, only for them to be very surprised to report that their pain has vanished, and often never to return.

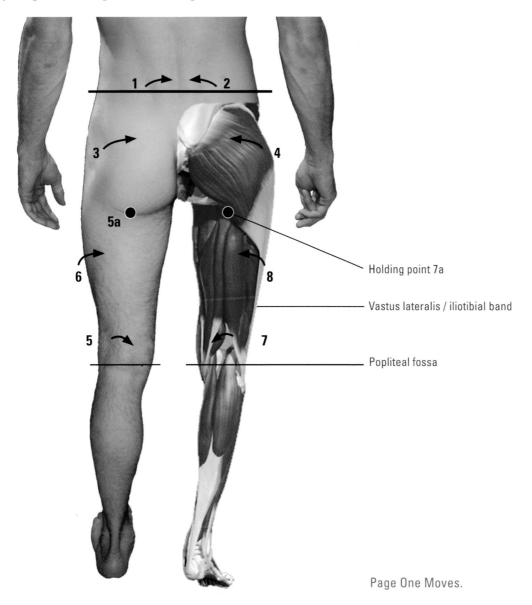

Holding point 7a

Vastus lateralis / iliotibial band

Popliteal fossa

Page One Moves.

The move itself needs to be performed slowly not only to line up the conjoined elements of the structures going into it, but also to get the right degree of pressure so as to make the HTL a rolling-type move rather than the 'clunk' that can easily happen if the move is made too quickly.

With the leg in extension and flat on the table, the patella should be able to move around reasonably freely over the knee. If it can't, the HTL move should free it up. If, however, the patella is still reluctant after a couple of goes, then gently moving it from side to side will help, thus freeing it up to track backwards and forwards across the knee joint.

The upper shoulder and neck represent a key area when addressing the posture and movement patterns of the body. The natural tendency for people to slightly raise their shoulder as a normal way of movement can create a great deal of tension in the area, and compensation for this will then be necessary elsewhere in the body.

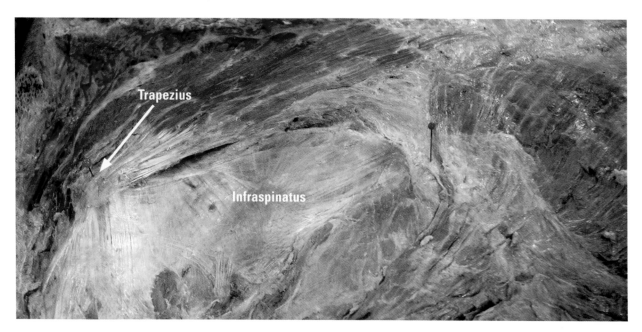

The fascia of the deltoid here blends seamlessly with that of the trapezius and infraspinatus.
Where does one begin to define muscle?

The connection of the levator scapulae to the superior medial angle of the scapula creates a tensional pull upwards into the neck and makes this small attachment point an area of concentrated fascial relationships. Although the deltoid is indicated as being attached to the lower lip of the spine of the scapula, we can see in the above illustration that the furthest medial aspects of it reach across to the superior medial angle and seem to blend in with the fascia of the trapezius. This creates tension laterally from the deltoid, medially from the trapezius and superiorly from the levator scapulae. No wonder people feel so much tension in this area.

In many cases clients reporting with 'neck pain' will put their hands over the top of this scapula region to indicate where the problem is. The pain will often radiate into the neck and back of the head, and this is a very classical indication of the scapula attachments being the culprit. The problem with this 'lifted scap' scenario is that, once the postural pattern has been established, collagen fibres come along to support this and create even more tension. In addition, the presentation of peripheral pains in the hands and arms can often be attributed to this slight raising of the scapula.

FROZEN SHOULDER

In the case of a 'frozen shoulder' the slight raising of the scapula will effectively 'lock' it into a semi-fixed position, thus preventing full range of movement of the arm. Exploration of the deltoid and upper arm might be necessary, but the area around the scapula needs to be taken care of first.

The upper body area can be looked at in much the same way as the pelvis. Elevation, rotation or winging of the scapula will have an effect somewhere else, often the mid-back or lower back, and usually on the opposite side. Whilst some of the more forward-thinking anatomical programmes and books will show some layers of fascia, this is frequently shown as a plain white sheet. In reality, the deep fascia lies along strong multidirectional planes, which will be accentuated by the day-to-day functional activities of the client. The latissimus dorsi muscle, for instance, again covered in a strong layer of fascia, reaches down to the top edge of the sacrum, but the fascia continues into the deep layers of the tissues of the gluteus muscle on the opposite side. So we can confidently state that the right gluteus maximus is connected, and therefore potentially in communication, with the left latissimus dorsi.

It makes sense. If you walk along a straight line and think about how one arm swings ahead as the opposite leg steps forward, we can understand that the movement of our limbs is always in diagonals. Similarly, the action of learning to crawl is one which not only starts to lay down the rules for future movement, but is also an important part of brain development (Bell and Fox 1997). Observe the movement of the arms and shoulders of a client when they walk. Many people presenting with neck or shoulder pain will walk with little or no upper body movement – this will translate into how the shoulder blades are held. On palpation this lack of movement will be evident when trying to move the scapula, which will often feel literally stuck down. The moves around the scapula should free it up and restore a degree of normal movement, but, as with the patella, don't be afraid to gently move it around to help it along.

Pages Two and Three are really only broken down because of the position of the client when the moves are made. In fact the moves of Page Two can't really be called shoulder moves any more than neck moves, and, conversely, the moves of Page Three cannot be considered to be solely neck moves. Page Two can be broken down into two sections: one where moves are performed above the stoppers, and the other where moves are made in the area between the lower and upper stoppers (see moves 11–14, page 55).

Like Page One, the moves on the upper part are performed over areas of stress loading, which are areas that have to carry a lot of weight or strain. In order to create the three sections of the body – lower, middle and upper – the upper stoppers consist of four moves rather than two. The upper curve of the thoracic spine again serves as the location for these stoppers (moves 1–4), as they are points of physical stress. In most people, a line across the body from the bottom of one shoulder blade to the bottom of the other will give the peak of the primary curve. However, the curve will be lower (or more rarely higher) in some people; in these cases it is the peak of the curve that will be the reference point. In this area the erector spinae muscles are overlaid with less superficial fascia and are more liable to flick, so care should be taken to adjust the pressure used to make these four moves.

Moves 5–8 proceed around the rhomboid major and rhomboid minor, and drop over the levator scapulae. These moves aim to create more freedom of movement between the scapula and the spine, and between the scapula and the neck. The moves over the levator scapulae are referred to as 'ladybirds' because of the gruesome analogy of crushing a ladybird under your thumb. It is important to understand where the medial border and the spine of the shoulder blade are located. Take some time to palpate the scapula, and work with a skeleton model to familiarise yourself with the various features of the scapula, in particular the spine and the superior medial angle and how it forms the acromion. It is important not to cut off the corner of the scapula but instead use the whole surface of the thumb to roll around it. The clicking feeling of the ladybird is the conjunction of the fascia of several muscle groups, but sometimes a clicking can also be felt when cutting the corner, so care needs to be taken here.

The section sitting above the spine of the scapula houses the supraspinatus, an interesting muscle and a really important aspect of arm movement. It is an area I will work with at various times, but for the moment we need to stay directly away from it. Fascially it links into the rhomboids and has the trapezius sitting on top of it, so they all play a role in shoulder and arm function.

Most muscle charts illustrate the trapezius as being separate from the deltoid, with the deltoid attaching to the upper part of the spine of the scapula. As you can see from the following picture, the deltoid in fact appears to be continuing into the fascia of the upper trapezius. With the levator scapulae sitting underneath this arrangement, you can see why any attempt to address the shoulder and neck needs to be referenced from this junction.

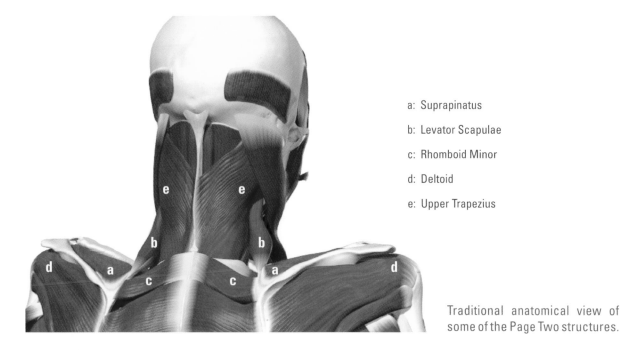

a: Suprapinatus

b: Levator Scapulae

c: Rhomboid Minor

d: Deltoid

e: Upper Trapezius

Traditional anatomical view of some of the Page Two structures.

The location for moves 9 and 10 can be found on a line lateral to the bottom edge of the shoulder blade. If you keep below this line, any move you make will always be over the latissimus dorsi. Going above the line, however, introduces the possibility of the move being made over the teres major instead. The latissimus dorsi brings us face to face with the complex nature of where parts of the upper body become parts of the lower body. The muscle descends obliquely down to the lower back, where it blends into the fascia of the sacrum and becomes part of the complex structure known as the thoracolumbar fascia. This area, which will be discussed in greater detail later in the book, is an area of multiple layers of fascia, blending into each other to create an incredibly dense, complex and multidirectional region, seemingly acting as some kind of biomechanical fuse box for the rest of the body.

At the junction of the shoulder blades, the latissimus dorsi twists slightly before heading to its attachment site on the humerus, and is therefore much easier to locate. The skin slack at this point should be taken very gently and carefully. The muscle, being flaccid and relaxed, will be easily pushed out of the way by excessive pressure, making the muscle itself hard to locate and roll over. There is also the additional element of a lot of lymph nodes in this location – something to consider as part of a lymphatic treatment. At this point it is easy to end up too high on the lateral portion of the shoulder blade, picking up along the way the teres major and minor. Of course, this isn't going to be harmful; in fact, it is an area that we need to consider for more chronic shoulder problems. However, in terms of connecting, treatment of this area doesn't have the same impact as working the latissimus dorsi, and so we should make the effort to get the location right.

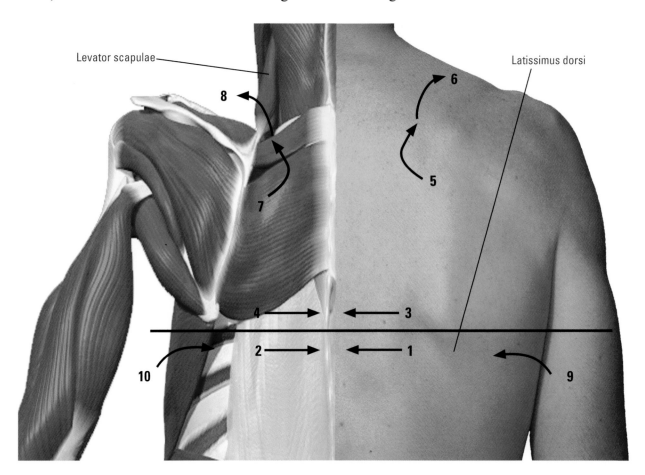

Moves 11–14 are used to work the midsection of the back, which can often be difficult to address. The spinal root nerves of this area relate to many digestive and organic functions, and these moves are useful as a starting point for these conditions. We can think of these moves as laces, going from one side of the body to the other, performing medial and lateral moves along the erector spinae. I have already mentioned the idea of moves along the spine being in different directions for different reasons. As far as it seems plausible, the medial moves along the erector spinae appear to create an opening effect – a release of tension and rigidity. On the other hand, the lateral moves along the erector spinae seem to create a drawing in and energising effect, creating tone and integrity in flaccid or tired structures.

It does seem like quite a lot of work is involved, and in many ways there is. As a student progresses, he or she learns that most of these moves are optional, and defined only by the needs of the client. We can stop at any stage, even if it is just for a few minutes, to see whether, on returning, there has been sufficient change to allow us to stop the treatment.

CHAPTER 7

Page Three

As mentioned earlier, Page Two and Page Three are considered to be procedures that will generally be performed together. There is no real separation between what we refer to as the neck and the shoulders, and it is impossible to say exactly where one begins and the other ends. The levator scapulae, for instance, is a muscle that is very often associated with neck pain, attaching as it does to the neck in a four-fingered formation, but also attaching to the top inside edge of the shoulder blade. So, neck or shoulder?

The human head weighs in the region of 14 lbs, or just over 6 kg, and sits forward of the rest of the spine, reflecting the natural state of being slightly flexed in an upright position. With the head weighing so much, the muscular requirements of the neck are many fold, and there is a great need for stability in the presence of such potential strain.

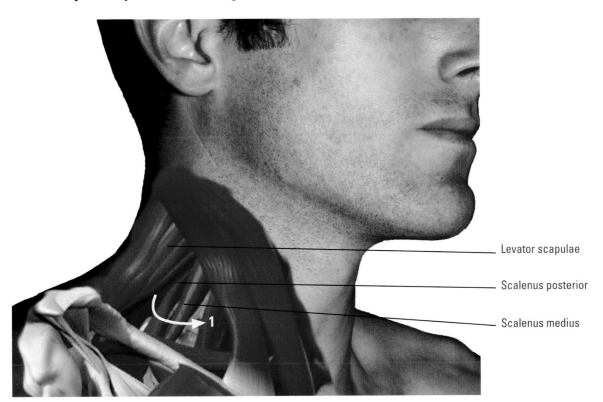

Levator scapulae

Scalenus posterior

Scalenus medius

The first moves of Page Three, moves 1 and 2, around the base of the neck, need to be far enough posteriorly to also pick up the mid-portion of the levator scapulae where they come under and in front of the trapezius. A rolling move with the thumbs will then pick up the scalenes – an important group of structures in the neck that not only give movement to both the head and the neck, but also help to lift the ribcage in their role as accessory muscles of respiration.

It is important to get far enough back in order to allow the thumb to roll all the way around the base of the neck. This means that the thumb should be kept straight rather than bent, and it is necessary to wait until the webbing of the hand is almost all the way around the neck before the thumb makes its move. The hollow at the base of the neck is just in front of the trapezius and forms a perfect dip for the thumb to fit into. There really isn't any skin slack available here; instead, the action of pushing the thumb into this small depression takes the skin back and creates the space for the thumb to move around.

Moves 3 and 4 are very small but powerful, reaching right up into the back of the head onto a couple of small muscles – the spinalis capitis and the semispinalis capitis. These muscles usually blend into each other, and are responsible for the holding of the head up. In addition, the greater occipital nerve passes between them; trapping or putting pressure on this nerve is responsible for a whole host of neck and head pains, so it is important to be in the right place when doing these moves.

An error that a lot of people make is to come down along the occipital ridge to make these moves. The main reason for doing this is that there isn't much of a move to make here, and the temptation is always to look for something more palpable to move over. The reference point of the occipital protuberance is an important one, as this gives us a clearer location for the move. It is generally a point at which there is always a degree of tenderness, and which, if worked accurately, can lead to remarkable release for headaches and tension. There's no need to go in with much pressure here.

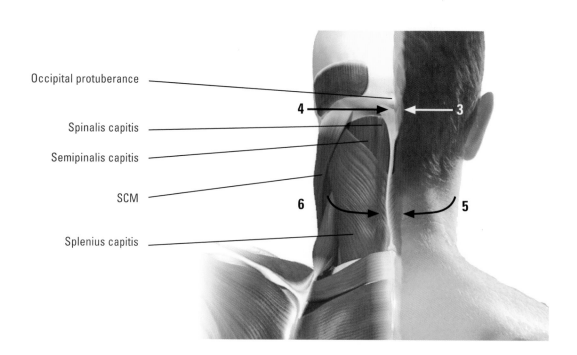

Occipital protuberance

Spinalis capitis

Semipinalis capitis

SCM

Splenius capitis

The move itself is very small and doesn't feel particularly satisfactory. All you can really feel here is hair, skin and what feels like bone. Yet the tenderness of the area belies the level of structural tension held here, and even the smallest move will have a dramatic effect. This is an area which needs to be considered in virtually every presentation, even the lower back. The position of the head and its relationship to the rest of the spine means that huge pressures and tensions are stored in this small area. The rest of the fascia of the head starts to join up here, and other major muscle groups, such as the sternocleidomastoid (SCM), connect fascially to this strong bony area. So the move may be small, but the power and effect shouldn't be underestimated. As well as the neck and shoulder presentations that we would expect to explore by working this point, we should also consider this point whenever there are upper limb, arm, wrist or hand problems. Again, the position of the head is hugely relevant to the strain that is being experienced in the neck. Excessive tension and strain ensure that the neck will take on the load and create potential follow-on strain through to the arms and hands. Structural tension in the body can never be experienced in isolation, but instead has to have some kind of compensation elsewhere. It is this compensation that causes the conflict which we may experience as stiffness, aching or soreness, and which creates the potential for damage.

Although a two-minute break is indicated after moves 3 and 4, I always recommend that the duration is extended to around four or five minutes. I would also consider going back to the moves if a lot of tension or tenderness is present. This location is a very useful barometer of the tensional state of the head and neck, but should not be over-handled.

On a recent skiing holiday I was careless enough to experience a heavy fall, my skis flying out from underneath me and the back of my head cracking onto an icy patch lurking underneath the snow. It was quite a violent head blow and one of the worst I have ever experienced, but fortunately I was wearing a helmet. Shaken, but otherwise unhurt, I continued to ski. The next day I awoke with a stiff neck that continued to develop over the next four days. Every movement, especially lifting my head from the pillow, was painful and an effort. A long-standing expert on neck pain, I found that this was different, as the pain didn't stem from the usual area at the back of the shoulder, but was concentrated in the front of the neck around the SCM. It was a superb opportunity to see at first hand the effect of a forced impact to the back of the head, resulting in a whiplash effect on the anterior portion of my neck and head. The pain even radiated into the upper chest for some time.

Finally, moves 5 and 6 of Page Three are over the trapezius, but also over the underlying splenius capitis. The latter muscle works with the SCM to put the head and neck into lateral flexion, and also shares an attachment site with the SCM on the mastoid process of the temporal bone. Together with the posterior belly of the digastric muscle, a three-way tensional marriage takes place, with the temporomandibular joint (TMJ) sitting in the middle of it all. These moves are a classic Bowen-type roll, and care should be taken to avoid flicking the muscle. A lot of information about the tone of the neck can be obtained here, and it is a place where over-manipulation with high-velocity thrust techniques or poor muscle tone can be easily picked up on.

From this working position it is also useful to quickly scan down the body, checking the position of the head in relation to the shoulders and the rest of the body down through to the feet. Also, looking down from the head of the client, the pelvis can often be observed to be rotated or tilted, leading you to perform a more thorough investigation. It is not unusual for the neck to change quite quickly with the set moves performed around it, and, on sitting the client up, care should be taken to make sure that they are not light-headed afterwards.

There has been much discussion as to whether moves 5 and 6 can or should be repeated. Whilst I personally have no problem with the occasional move being repeated, it is worth being mindful of any routines or habits that can be set up. I therefore advise avoiding repeating moves unless there is clear motivation and reasoning for doing so which could be justified. Simply putting in more moves because one can is retrograde, rarely has much useful function, and generally leads to the hard-to-break habit of arbitrarily repeating moves.

Pages One, Two and Three create a remarkable balance throughout the body and in most instances are more than enough for a first treatment. The mistake we all make is to go through these procedures as a monotonous routine: first four moves, take a break, second four moves, take a break, and so forth. This is an opportunity missed. The amount of information transmitted and received during these procedures is immense, and the ability to vary the order and direction of the moves means that there are literally millions of potential variations. The moves themselves cover most of the highly stress-loaded areas of the human form; if applied with care and concentration, they can often be reduced to a series of 10 or 12 moves, making an entire and profound treatment.

Because most of the moves are performed on the back of the client, it follows that there will tend to be a greater concentration of superficial adipose tissue, so the need for skilful palpation comes to the fore. Yet even the newest of students will attain impressive and rapid responses from these initial procedures. I spend much of my time reading case histories submitted by students, always being amazed at the responses that Pages One to Three elicit. There is much more to discover around the neck and the head, particularly the connecting relationships further down into the body, around to the chest and across into the arms. But for the moment, getting these amazing moves right is task enough!

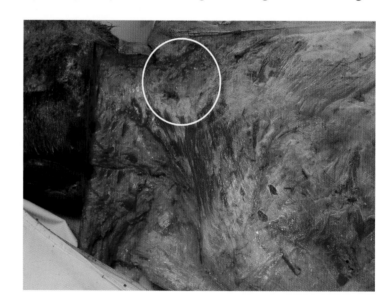

The continuous nature of the neck and shoulder tissues is shown in this picture.

Note the thickness of the skin around the neck area and the build-up of sinewy, fatty deposits around the base of the neck. This suggests a position with the head being held forwards, a common tendency in the elderly. It is hard to differentiate muscles from each other in this area, and the image clearly demonstrates how divisions between areas we refer to as neck or shoulder are arbitrary when it comes to connective tissue.

BACK TO BASICS?

I have spent many years being incredibly familiar with Pages One to Three of Bowen Therapy, and given treatment and taught these moves to thousands of people. Considering that I generally have the attention span of a five-year-old, I am amazed at my sticking power and fascination with this simple set of gentle moves. One part of my job is marking the case histories that students send in after they have completed the initial stages of their training, which includes the learning of Pages One to Three. Whilst sometimes the job can be a chore, it is transformed by the constant amazement that I have on seeing the results that people get using this 'basic' work. How does it do what it does? In spite of a section in this book, I truly have no idea. Yet something very powerful is going on.

Then comes the time when people want more, and the tendency for these moves to become automatic or routine creeps in. No longer are we thinking about what we are doing, or trying to feel what is happening. Instead we are putting in the moves and thinking about what we are having for tea. I see people on workshops who are belting through these moves, in a hurry to get them out of the way and move on to more and more procedures, more learning, more moves. Yet the variety of ways in which these moves can be applied is almost infinite. Once the stoppers have been put in, you can go anywhere on the body to link up one move to another.

For those of you that have perhaps forgotten the power of this initial work, I encourage you to experiment with what you have in Pages One to Three. Slow down the move, lighten your touch, mix up the order, or simply concentrate on what you are doing and feel the changes under your fingers. These are not basic moves: these are a work of genius. I fall in love with them and the effect they have, every day.

In the next few chapters, I am going to wander through the rest of the classical Bowen repertoire, giving no order in terms of importance, but simply working in alphabetical order.

CHAPTER 8

Ankle

The ankle is one of the procedures often forgotten in the normal run of things. Unless a client is presenting with some kind of ankle pain or problem, many therapists simply don't use these moves. This is a shame, as the ankle procedure is a key move for addressing the posture of the whole body. The foot contains 26 bones, all of which are connected by a series of ligaments and tendons to the rest of the leg. The bones of the foot move and create flexibility, but they also dictate where the pressure for the rest of the leg, the hip and the back will come from.

"The foot is the conductor of the body's muscular orchestra. They all pay attention to his movements and follow where he leads them."

The ankle is the set-up or precursor for each step that we take. Putting pressure onto the foot pre-warns the hip, lower back and shoulders to contract or to move in a certain direction. If any kind of physiological feedback loop suggests that this will be difficult or painful, then the changes in the step will reflect this, resulting in the step having a different pressure and emphasis. Recent fascial studies have framed the fascia as a sort of feed-forward mechanism – tissue which in some way seems to set up the rest of the body for what is about to happen.

The connection upwards through the body is mediated through the sacrum, which seems to act as a type of fuse box for the muscular structures coming to it and going from it. The first move, across the extensor retinaculum, is worth exploring, as it is a classic example of traditional anatomy not entirely giving the whole picture. In most anatomy books we will see the extensor retinaculum as a quite distinct section of fascia, wrapping around the ankle. In fact the image (overleaf) that we see is what is left behind when the rest of the fascial covering of the leg is removed. This fascia – the fascia lata, meaning white fascia – is a continuous sheet of fascia that blends upwards into the iliotibial band and around the rest of the leg.

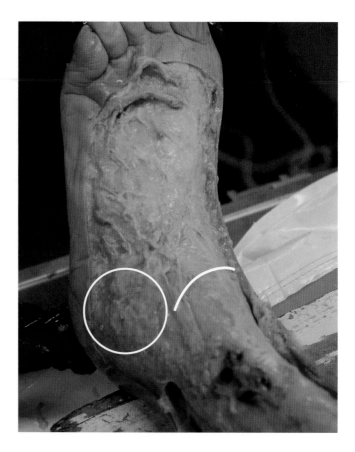

The extensor retinaculum is barely visible here, simply because it is still integral to the rest of the fascia of the leg. The circle indicates the approximate position of the lateral malleolus. As can be seen here, the concept of a retinaculum is questionable anyway (Marwan and Harris 2009).

We can therefore see a direct connection between the lateral move of the knee (see page 110) and the first ankle move. The retinaculum is simply a thicker part of this sock-like sheet, holding in place – like a piece of sticky tape – the three muscle groups that pass under it. However, these groups are also encased in their own sheaths, thereby allowing free movement of the fibres backwards and forwards through the sock.

The sock, as we can see, is a continuation of the tight ITB, which also blends in seamlessly below the knee with the fascia of the extensor digitorum longus. Although referred to as a muscle of the anterior compartment, the extensor digitorum longus – as shown by palpation – starts more laterally, as an extension of the ITB, before winding its way forwards to arrive at the front of the foot. Lateral knee pain therefore needs the ankle to be looked at, almost as a matter of course. If there is any kind of eversion or untoward movement through the foot, the biggest point of tensional resistance will be at this major junction at the lateral knee.

The first ankle move acts as an effective mediator between the foot and the rest of the leg, as the muscle group here refers to all the muscles of the anterior compartment of the leg. The tibialis anterior has a very long attachment to the tibia, although, as we have already explored in the myths section (see page 17), muscles don't really attach to bone in the way we have assumed. This dichotomy is an important one here, as certain conditions of the leg can be more easily explained if we understand this relationship. The long attachment of the tibialis anterior is wrapped in a thin layer of fascia, which in turn attaches to the fascia of the tibial bone – the periosteum. If we imagine two surfaces attached to each other at one point, but with layers underneath that can ever so slightly rub and create friction, we can then understand how inflammation can occur.

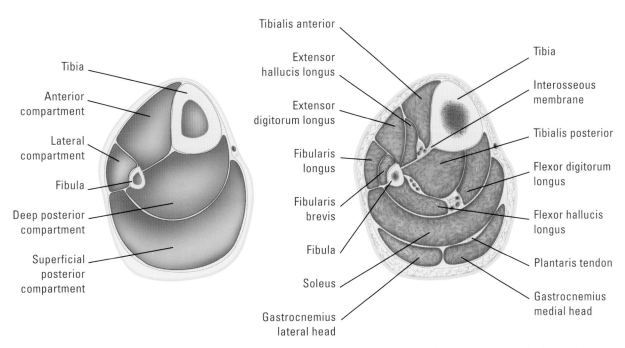

Tibialis anterior

Extensor hallucis longus

Extensor digitorum longus

Fibularis longus

Fibularis brevis

Fibula

Soleus

Gastrocnemius lateral head

Tibia

Anterior compartment

Lateral compartment

Fibula

Deep posterior compartment

Superficial posterior compartment

Tibia

Interosseous membrane

Tibialis posterior

Flexor digitorum longus

Flexor hallucis longus

Plantaris tendon

Gastrocnemius medial head

Cross section of the lower leg.

Try this: put the palms of your hands together and without allowing the surface of the skin to slide around, move them against each other. You will feel slight movement under the skin and before long, heat will start to build up at the interface between your hands. If you translate this slight frictional rubbing into the shins, and imagine the number of times that this would happen as someone ran or jogged, then we can understand how anterior leg pain, sometimes called 'shin splints', can occur. In order to clarify this, we can therefore rename the condition to 'anterior tibial fasciitis' or 'inflammation of the anterior tibial fascia'. By working the interfaces where most of the tension lies, particularly across the muscle group where it passes under the retinaculum, we can address this type of problem effectively. However, further work along the surface of the tibia might also be required in some instances.

The second move addresses the fibres of the fibularis longus and brevis muscles, which come from the posterior part of the calf. These strong bands are held in a tight groove around the back of the lateral ankle bone, and again need to slide in and out within this groove if the normal flexion and extension of the foot is to be achieved. The clearing action of this posterior move ensures that the follow-up move takes into account the full shape of both small muscular groupings and fascial groupings.

On the medial side, three strong ligaments – the tibiotalar, tibiocalcaneal and tibionavicular – emerge from the tibia to attach to the three corresponding bones of the foot, creating a tensional relationship between the leg and the foot. In addition, the flexor digitorum longus sits adjacent to the tibialis posterior, and is involved in plantar flexion of the foot, as well as working to keep us standing upright. If it is overly contracted or shortened, the result can be claw toes, although it is worth remembering that this muscle is also intimately involved with the soleus muscle at the back of the calf. The other player in this third ankle move is the tibialis posterior, coming around the back edge of the medial malleolus in another groove. The tibialis posterior plays a big role in stabilising the foot and is often indicated in flat feet, where the muscle is overly stretched. Again, as is always the case, these indications don't arise independently, and a good look to see what else is involved in the process will be required.

So, in three small moves, all the major muscular attachments of the leg and the foot are addressed, before the foot is then effectively reset between the tibia and fibula bones of the leg by the push. The push will also have a releasing effect on the Achilles tendon and therefore potentially on pain found in the sole of the foot. If the foot is positioned correctly, then forward movement will be in balance, and unequal pressure on the rest of the lower body will be avoided. From a fascial perspective, the fascia of the front and back of the foot rise clearly upwards into the back and abdomen, and beyond.

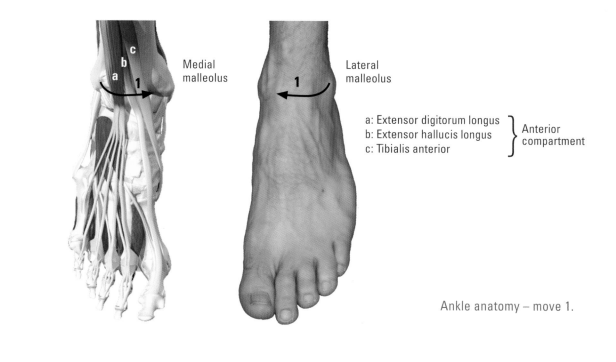

Medial
malleolus

Lateral
malleolus

a: Extensor digitorum longus
b: Extensor hallucis longus   } Anterior
c: Tibialis anterior   compartment

Ankle anatomy – move 1.

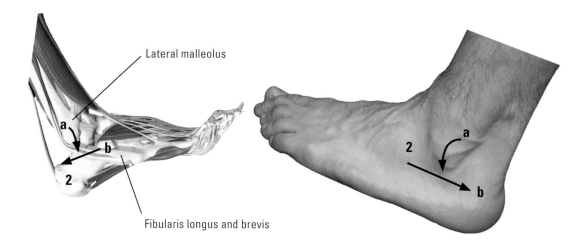

Lateral malleolus

Fibularis longus and brevis

Ankle anatomy – move 2.

The minimum prerequisite for the ankle is to 'hit the lats', but wherever possible, Page One should also be used in order to establish a good balance and to cover other eventualities. It is also important to not just think of the ankle locally: a non-responding ankle or foot will need the lower back, pelvis and gluteal areas addressed.

Take some time to look at the position of the feet in relation to the legs and the rest of the body. Consider whether, like the tyres on a car, there is more 'wear' on one side or the other, which might suggest imbalance. A good indication would be a build-up of excess skin around the heels or toes. You can also consider the position of one foot compared to the other, when the client is lying face up. Does one foot sit in a different position, point in a different direction or appear to have a different shape? These assessments are not made in order to determine what, if anything, is wrong, or to make a diagnosis, but simply in order to be able to ask questions, gather information and compare any changes from week to week.

As well as following the muscle groupings of the leg downwards, work being performed at the lower end will also have an effect through the knee, and the ankle should be seen as an extension of the knee and hamstring procedures. In conclusion, the ankle procedure, particularly in conjunction with the pelvis procedure (see page 115), can be used for a whole range of presentations and is not limited to problems of the foot and ankle. That said, it is also very useful for the treatment of acute ankle problems and sports injuries, and should be used in conjunction with the remedies for reducing inflammation and swelling.

Most of the time we will generally perform moves on the better side where one exists; an exception would be the case of an acute ankle strain. As I have suggested previously, the body is set for a touch response when the better side is treated first. If the client has already seen what you intend to do by your having done the better side first, the prospect of a sharp push onto a painful ankle may well worry or stress the client, causing reluctance or fear of this being done.

There is one slight caveat to this whole treatment in the case where the client experiences sharp pain when their ankle is handled. There are occasions where, even when an X-ray has been taken, fractures have been missed. The ankle and foot is a complex structure, so if in any doubt, stop the treatment and refer the client to the nearest emergency department or doctor's surgery. Better safe than sued!

CHAPTER 9

Breast

Firstly, in spite of the name of the procedure, we must be clear that this procedure does not involve any work on what might be considered breast tissue. We are instead dealing with the structures immediately above and below the tissues, aiming to affect the muscular and lymphatic tissues associated with it.

Breast cancer is one of the most common cancers in the UK, although as a percentage of all cancers, the number of cases is still relatively small. The increase over the years has been blamed on numerous things, and the conventional response has been limited and somewhat ineffective. Suggested factors contributing to breast cancer include underwired bras, electromagnetic radiation, sugar intake, hormone replacement, lack of exercise, food allergies and production, and underarm deodorant, to name a few. Whilst none of these have been shown to conclusively cause cancer, there are many questions which still need answering. The conventional response has been to promote mammography as a preventative measure. However, there is still a great deal of academic debate as to the effectiveness of this approach, with some suggestion that it does not effectively reduce the incidence of breast cancer.

As a matter of common sense, however, we can see that there are some measures that women can take in order limit congestion in the breast area. Underwired bras create a level of restriction in this area, which will undoubtedly lead to a slow down of lymphatic movement. Quite apart from anything else, many women will be wearing ill-fitting bras that will only increase the problem. The answer here is to encourage as much 'wire-free' time as possible, along with measures such as body brushing to encourage movement of lymph and removal of dead surface skin cells.

Where hormonal issues are present, the breast procedure is also indicated as an assistant for procedures such as the coccyx. The breast tissue is home to a lot of hormonal activity, especially those concerning menstruation and breast-feeding. From a structural perspective, the breast move works with the pectoralis major, which is in continuity with the deltoid as well as with itself at the front. It can therefore be seen as a useful addition to the shoulder procedure.

The area of the first move – the pectoralis – is continuous, as a structure, with the deltoid; separation of these can really only be achieved by cutting them apart. The second move is over the serratus anterior – a muscle which comes from the medial side of the scapula. This muscle also helps to lift the ribs and so can be seen as part of the process of respiration, making this procedure a useful add-on to any diaphragmatic presentation.

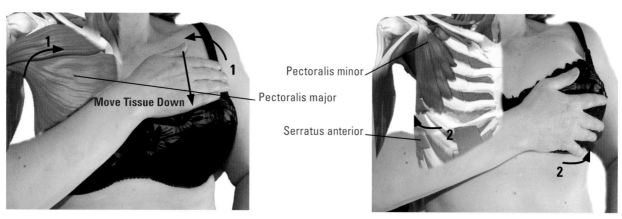

Breast procedure – move 1.

Breast procedure – move 2.

LYMPHATICS

The lymphatic system is part of the circulatory system. It comprises a network of channels, lymphatic vessels, nodes and ducts that collect and carry a clear fluid called lymph.

The lymphatic system has several important functions:

- Transporting fatty acids and fats from the digestive system.

- Working with the immune system to fight infection.

- Maintaining the body's fluid balance.

- Transporting white blood cells to and from the lymph nodes and the bones.

In addition to lymph nodes, lymphatic tissues are also present in lymphoid organs. These tissues assist the lymphatic system and include the appendix, spleen, thymus and tonsils as well as specialised tissues in the small intestine.

The lymphatic system doesn't have a single method of movement: it relies instead on already existing functions, in particular muscular contraction, for the transportation of lymph around the body. As a result, concentrations of nodes will be found in areas where there is likely to be substantial movement, although lymph nodes can be found almost anywhere.

The Bowen lymphatic procedures target the areas in which these concentrations of nodes are found:

- TMJ (SCM drainage). There are a lot of lymph nodes around the SCM, since this muscle is involved in most of the movements of the neck and head.

- Pelvis (Pelvic Procedure). The groin area along the line of the inguinal ligament is not only a site of movement, but also composed of several sheets of muscle and fascia of the abdomen.

- Breast (Breast Procedure). The breast area has a large concentration of lymph nodes. If bras were not used, this area would be very mobile, with the shoulder also contributing to movement as the most mobile joint of the body. The lack of shoulder movement, and in turn neck movement, could be a contributing factor in poor upper body lymphatic function.

- Kidney. Ultimately, the circulatory aspect of the lymphatic system relies heavily on effective filtration of blood and fluids. The kidney is therefore an important element.

The diaphragm is also heavily indicated in lymphatic function. Around the thoracic area there is a concentration of lymph nodes which will be affected by a change in respiration. However, because these are not in an area which is touched on directly by the Bowen procedure, we would not include them in a list of lymphatic procedures.

Similarly, although the knee around the popliteal fossa and the calf would be part of the process of lymph drainage, these areas would be worked as part of the prerequisite procedures for the pelvis.

As mentioned earlier, body movement is a key element in good lymphatic function. Encouraging our clients to walk and move as much as possible will be an important factor in aftercare as well as in addressing long-term issues, including immune system weakness and dysfunction.

As we have already mentioned lymph, we can include the breast procedure as one of the four specific procedures which address the lymphatic system. The breast tissue and surrounding areas are host to a lot of lymphatic vessels, and the nature of the breast tissue area is very wet and fatty. Circulation in this area is therefore vital. Of course, we see the breasts and their circulation as mostly a female issue, but the presence of lymph nodes and the need for this area to be moved is not restricted to women.

It's no accident that an area rich in lymph nodes, which require muscular contraction for them to be squeezed and to do their job, is located around the most mobile joint in the body – the shoulder. The idea would therefore be that lots of movement of the shoulder will promote the movement of lymph through the upper body. Moreover, this shoulder movement would also promote an increase in respiratory function, driving the lymph nodes in the thoracic cavity as well. It is therefore something of an irony that – as well as not climbing trees or throwing things, which would be a good workout for our shoulders and our respiratory system – we actively promote the use of clothing that will severely restrict what natural flow there is.

The second move will require the client to lift the breast tissue up. If the client is wearing an underwired bra, they should put their little finger under the wire in order to prevent pressure being put onto the breast tissue by the wire in the bra. Consequently, if this move is performed correctly, there is no direct contact of the therapist with breast tissue at all, and the procedure should not feel invasive or in any way inappropriate to either the therapist or client.

There has been discussion over the years about whether this procedure can be applied in situations where there are breast implants or reconstructions. As with most cases, a degree of common sense needs to prevail here, and I am wary of a blanket ban. Women who have undergone reconstruction following mastectomies, particularly where the latissimus dorsi has been brought around, sometimes have restrictions and pain through the shoulder and back. Bowen in these cases can be very beneficial, but it is always worth discussing things carefully with the client.

Breast implants have had a history of failures, such as the implant leaking or presenting problems. More recently, issues have arisen where the content of the implant has been questionable, and patients have taken legal action. In these instances, information about other treatments will be sought as part of the legal process; treatments undertaken on or near the breast area could be cited as being reasons for the problems, bringing the process into question. In these unusual and rare circumstances, it has therefore been suggested that the breast procedure should be avoided. However, this is not to suggest or imply that the procedure is in any way dangerous or contraindicated where breast implants are present. In fact, there are many good reasons why this procedure would be very helpful and indicated where surgery has taken place.

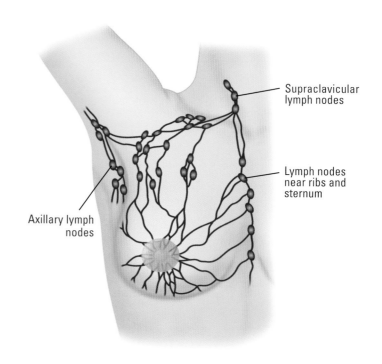

Supraclavicular lymph nodes

Lymph nodes near ribs and sternum

Axillary lymph nodes

Breast procedure.

CAUTION

This move does not require the removal or adjustment of underwear or light clothing. Ensure that you discuss this procedure with your client before proceeding and have a third party present if necessary. Be clear about your level of communication, and ask questions from the perspective of the client, noting carefully not only the verbal aspect of all communication, but also how someone comes across when you are talking to them. Checking with the client that they truly are comfortable will have the effect of making them comfortable.

CHAPTER 10

Coccyx

One of the smallest and most straightforward in the Bowen repertoire, the coccyx move gets to the very heart of many issues which present in doctors' surgeries as well as to complementary therapists all over the country.

Stress is a regularly used word (sometimes too much) by people day in and day out to describe the physical and emotional pressures that surround their daily lives. Pressures of work, money, relationships, teenagers, parking spaces, neighbours – you name it, and someone somewhere will be getting stressed about it. Yet what does this word mean? If we think about structures such as bridges or struts under stress, they are being exposed to such pressures that, without additional support or strength, will cause them to ultimately collapse. We could apply the same reasoning to the human condition. A pressurised job might be one in which there is a call to perform at a certain level. As long

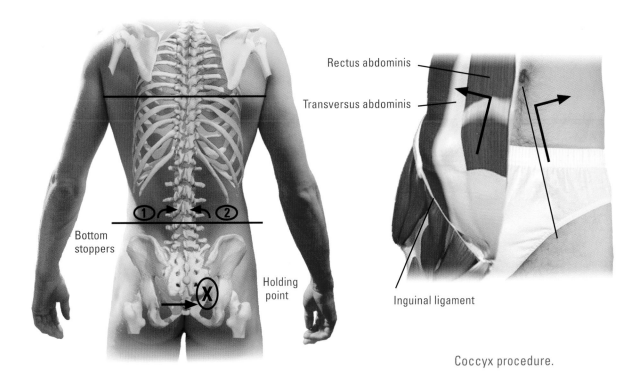

Coccyx procedure.

as all the supporting structures are in place, such pressure might be highly enjoyable and motivating. However, with a shortage of staff and resources to do the job effectively, the same pressures will become massively stressful.

The autonomic nervous system (ANS) has two branches: the sympathetic nervous system (SNS) and the parasympathetic nervous system (PNS). The system which mediates the stress response – the SNS – is vitally important and is in place as a life-saver. The SNS is often referred to as the fight-or-flight system and mediates rapid changes in the body's systems when immediate changes in energy requirements are called for.

If we were to encounter a grizzly bear on our trip to the local shop, we would need to quickly call on some resources to help us to deal with the situation. If we were going to run for it, we would need to access energy rapidly. This would come primarily from our digestive system, which consumes up to 25% of the body's energy at any one time. Our bowels might therefore be filled with fluid in order to get rid of undigested food, with the inevitable consequences! We would also need to divert blood to supply major muscle groups, take blood away from the skin and peripheral tissues (this will also help to control bleeding in the case of injury), and release adrenalin to kill any pain we might have and speed up our heart rate. We might also start to shut down our immune and reproductive systems, neither of which are needed for short-term survival but which consume much-needed energy resources.

With these changes in place, we can fight, run or generally try to deal with the local bear much more effectively, thus increasing our chances of survival. All well and good. If the source of our stress was less immediate, however, but none the less the cause of a great deal of emotional trauma, the symptoms might well be very similar. Anyone who is experiencing what they call stress might also suffer from indigestion, racing heart, frequent colds and infections (reduction in immune system response), loss of libido, pins and needles in the hands (lack of peripheral blood supply) and so forth.

Originating in the brain, sympathetic projections exit your spine and branch out to nearly every organ, blood vessel and sweat gland in your body. They even project to the ends of the tiny little muscles attached to hairs on your body. If you are truly terrified, your hair stands on end. Goosebumps result when the parts of your body are activated where those muscles exist but lack hairs attached to them.

We have already addressed the principle of the stoppers and their ability to store energy in areas of stress loading. The coccyx can also be included in this system of stress loading given that it is the point of fine balance for our pelvis, as well as being the attachment site for the muscles of the pelvic floor.

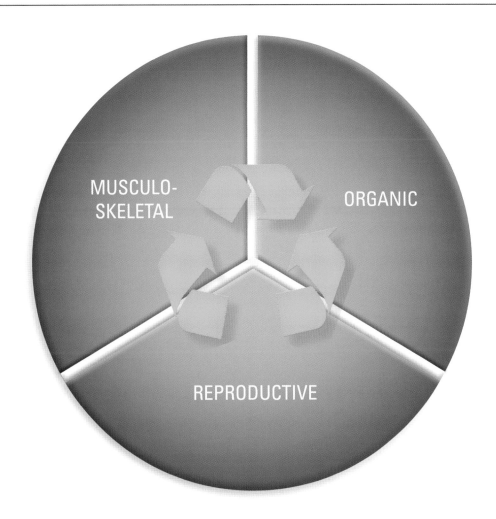

The coccyx can be broken down into three main areas of presentation which cover many of the three areas of concern. The pie chart illustrates this, with the arrows indicating that, although three sections have been drawn, they should not be regarded as separate areas but as parts of the whole system.

MUSCULOSKELETAL CONSIDERATIONS

From a musculoskeletal perspective the coccyx is the anchor point for the pelvic floor: the muscles of the pelvic floor all attach to, or have a strong fascial relationship with, the coccyx. This will mean that any issues relating to the pelvic floor would be addressed within the confines of this procedure. It is worth remembering that the male pelvic floor has the same muscular make-up as that of a female. However, the considerations of the vagina, combined with those of childbirth, tend to make the female pelvic floor more of an issue. In the male, the pelvic floor muscles will contribute to the function of the bladder and, in turn, the prostate and the erectile function of the penis.

The coccyx can also be considered a balancing point for the lower body – a kind of pendulum to determine how the rest of the spinal column will position itself. Fascially, the connections through the lower back are even more important. The thoracolumbar fascia blends into the coccyx and sacrum, linking up with the fascia of the pelvic floor and, in the female, the reproductive system; all these are held in place by strong fascial connections to the back of the coccyx and sacrum.

At the front, the muscles of the rectus abdominis descend to attach to the front of the pelvis at the pubic bone, again creating a clear continuity into the coccyx. The names of the muscles of the pelvic floor are, in themselves, a clue: coccygeus, pubococcygeus, iliococcygeus and so forth.

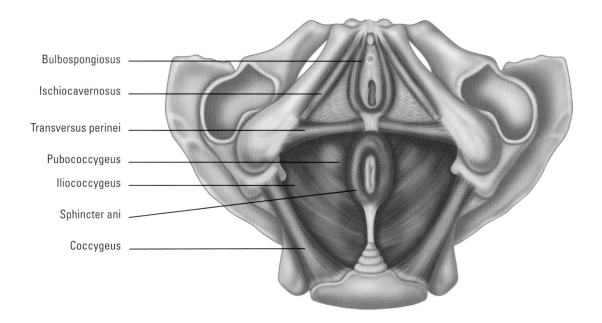

Bulbospongiosus

Ischiocavernosus

Transversus perinei

Pubococcygeus

Iliococcygeus

Sphincter ani

Coccygeus

ORGANIC FUNCTION

We have already referred to the SNS and the process of fight or flight that stimulation of the SNS engenders. In order to facilitate the functions required, the SNS will inhibit digestion. An example of continuous stress is the one witnessed in those with skin conditions such as psoriasis and eczema. Any of these sufferers will tell you that their symptoms are exacerbated by 'stress'. The skin, being the biggest organ of the body, can be seen as a barometer of many of the internal organs. Following Gil Hedley's presentation of the 'Onion Tree Model' of the body, all the organs of the body perforate the skin (Hedley 2007). Deane Juhan (2003), in *Job's Body*, refers to the skin as the surface of the brain, and goes on to say: "Its sensory pathways unite the surface and the interior of the organism, and its surface does not shield any more than it exposes."

Organically, therefore, the coccyx move aims to address and normalise organic function, including the peristaltic action of the colon. This is not likely to be addressed by the direct application of a very gentle move over the coccyx, but as a result of addressing the ANS. To this end we can use the coccyx to balance presenting conditions that are exacerbated by the existence of stress factors affecting the client. However, we need to carefully consider the meaning of this much overused word, and investigate what is meant by it. In engineering terms stress would refer to pressure on a structure which has insufficient strength to maintain it. The same definition could be applied to a human condition: lots of pressure and no effective support network. It could be a parent overwhelmed by responsibility and workload, and unsupported by their partner. Or perhaps an employee pressurised by unrealistic targets and given little in the way of support or effective training. We need to find out and give the client an opportunity to hear for themselves what the determining factor is. A simple question to ask, without the need for too much detail, could be: "What do you mean by 'stress'?"

REPRODUCTIVE ISSUES

In this section, the coccyx is considered to have two parts. The first part spills over into the musculoskeletal element, so the pelvic floor is addressed by the associated move. This applies to both male and female issues. In childbirth, the coccyx moves quite some way, and ideally this should not happen too quickly. If it does, then the potential for trauma and pelvic floor problems increases. A problem for some couples is the inability to conceive, or the inability for a woman to carry a baby to term. Little work or research has been done on the biomechanical reasons or treatments for these problems, yet it stands to reason that structural imbalances could easily play a key role.

The second part is, again, the involvement of the SNS, which will inhibit the body's reproductive capacity at times of stress. A good example of this is the stress and pressure which is put on a couple trying to conceive. There are many stories of couples conceiving naturally soon after adopting children. This suggests that perhaps the stress and pressure of trying to conceive paradoxically inhibited their natural ability to do so. Other factors are important here, including diet, alcohol and smoking, as well as the need for the testicles to be kept cooler than the rest of the body. Space, time and relevance to subject unfortunately prevent any great excursions into this topic right now.

In other issues surrounding the reproductive system, menopausal women presenting with hot flushes can be consistently helped with a variation of the coccyx procedure, which, for the most part, dissipate within one treatment.

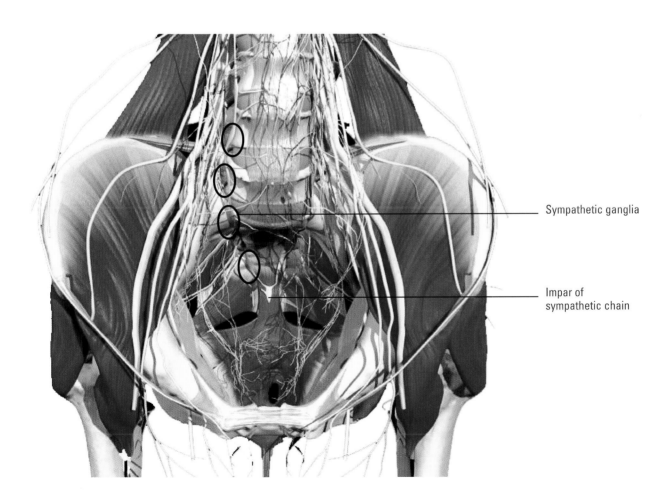

Sympathetic ganglia

Impar of sympathetic chain

THE OUTER CIRCLE

The pretty pie chart on page 75 is missing one vital component, mainly because the graphics would be spoiled. To this chart an outer circle could be added, which would then be labelled 'emotional' or 'mental'. This is sort of what I have been trying to get at when explaining the three sections. We are aiming for balance where imbalance exists. In the context of the coccyx, the imbalance is more likely to be there as a result of emotional or mental stress factors, which in turn have had knock-on effects on the body as a whole in any or all of the areas already mentioned. I would refer you to the excellent *Why Zebras Don't Get Ulcer*s by Robert Sapolsky (2004), for a more in-depth, but none the less very easy to understand, explanation of this subject.

APPLICATION

The move itself is made over the area where the sacrum and the coccyx join; this junction can be felt as a small knuckle of bone just down into the gluteal crease. It should be noted that we are not touching the end of the coccyx bone. Not only would that involve delving well down the crease and be invasive, but it would also be very painful for most people.

Although the move is made over the bone, it is still a skin move and very gentle. The holding point is effectively anywhere along the edge of the sacrum; it is made to stabilise the sacrum, whilst the leg being lifted allows the release of the ganglion impar (impar means 'unpaired') as well as providing more effective access to the area being worked. The holding point allows us to contain the release of the highly charged coccyx into the sacral area, before the second move subsequently uses this and carries it up into the rest of the body. Having the elbow pointed towards the head will allow the holding point to be kept still.

The sympathetic chain descends along the dorsal part of the spine, with fibrous branches going from small lumps or ganglia which sit alongside the rest of the nervous system and take part in regulating the ANS. At the time of need, these post-ganglionic fibres help to push the body into the stress response, which could be a life-saver. At the bottom of the chain, they join up at the ganglion impar. Because there is just one ganglion impar, only one move needs to be made over the coccyx, after having first assessed which side, if any, is the problem side. The assessment is less important than many people realise, but it does give the opportunity to palpate and ask questions. For the most part, skilled visual assessment will be enough, and paying attention to moves which have been made previously, especially moves 3 and 4 of Page One, will help us to build a picture of where tightness or tension is being held.

The coccyx move is traditionally seen as the last move performed on the client when they are prone, since a standard coccyx move is performed in this position. However, there are countless potential variations of this procedure, where the coccyx can be moved on both sides, with moves on the lumbar following on from the release of the coccyx. Remember, these are not advanced Bowen moves, as there is no such thing, but merely ways of working the body within the concept of Bowen, according to how one effectively reads the body and how one understands the effects of the work being used.

The move on the abdominal area is an interesting one, and something which I personally have questioned over the years. More understanding of what is being worked has come from dissective investigation. From this I have begun to understand the wrapping nature of abdominal tissue and its strong relationship to the thoracolumbar fascia, or TLF for short. All the abdominal muscles end, in one way or another, with a fascial link to the sacrum and coccyx and the TLF. It is this TLF that seems to act as a mediator for movement and function throughout the body – a concept which we can keep returning to when trying to investigate Bowen-type movements all over the system; it is an area which can be seen as a type of physical fuse box.

The coccyx move on the back, therefore, links beautifully with the wrapping-paper image of the abdominal structures, bringing the intensely energetic release of the highly charged coccyx into the multilayered bag of the abdominal region. The deeper layers of this area are intimately connected both spinally and viscerally, crossing and attaching to the spinal fascia, and therefore the sympathetic chain, as well as dropping deeply into the peritoneal bag which contains our viscera. At the same time, this wrapping is also highly energetic. Consisting of many layers, it is highly mobile and flexible, with the ability to stretch and adjust according to an incredible variety of situations.

The moves on the front of the body following a coccyx move are again traditionally completed first, before any other procedures are started. As with the moves on the back, there are a lot of variations that can be explored, not least the strong energetic area where the abdomen attaches to the diaphragm.

COCCYX IN PREGNANCY

A strongly held view over the years in the Bowen world is that the coccyx move should not be performed in pregnancy. Some reasonably logical reasons have been put forward for this, namely that it stimulates the ANS and therefore potentially creates some kind of potential for a woman to miscarry. It is certainly a very energetic area, and whilst I would tend to err on the side of caution, it would be negligent of me not to discuss the myths surrounding this potential panic button.

Nothing I have read, heard, investigated or had explained to me gives me any sound scientific or even intuitive reason for considering the coccyx move to be a source of potential miscarriage. If anything, the opposite might well be the case. The coccyx, as discussed, is a balancer of the ANS and is not there to stimulate or otherwise agitate a female reproductive system. If stress is a major factor in a woman's ability to conceive, and the coccyx a potential remedy for this, then it can hardly be deemed reasonable to suggest that the coccyx might also create a potential miscarriage. However, as I have already suggested, it is wise to be cautious. A woman miscarrying after a coccyx procedure might ask the question whether the procedure had perhaps been a cause. My answer would be an emphatic no, but perhaps it would be better not to be put in that situation in the first place.

There are some very good reasons why a woman should be treated with a coccyx procedure during pregnancy, high blood pressure being one of them. However, I would suggest that it is not done until after the twelfth week of pregnancy, after which time I am totally convinced it could be performed by an experienced practitioner on a regular basis.

The make-up of the coccyx, together with the nature of what we are trying to achieve in this area, means that we need to proceed with some degree of caution. Communication is very important: we must explain carefully and thoroughly the process and location, and get clear consent. Although the move is not really near the anus, it is below the line of the pants and into the gluteal crease, and we should consider the emotional comfort of the client at all times. Again, because of the nature of the work, this is not a procedure which would be performed at a first treatment. We have only just met this client and have no idea how they will react to Bowen. In effect, we are strangers, and a coccyx procedure simply isn't going to be an appropriate first line of treatment. As with all the procedures at this level, we need to think about what is really needed and step back wherever possible.

The TMJ procedure (see page 140) is also something that we should avoid using in combination with the coccyx. As I explained earlier, we work with an area addressing the parasympathetic nervous system with the TMJ. Although our ultimate goal is the same, we need to be somewhat circumspect in how we get there.

BEDWETTING

A child over the age of six or seven who is wetting the bed on a regular basis could benefit from a variation of the coccyx procedure. Under this age, I consider that children are little more than babies, and would be a little concerned by a parent feeling that a young child should be pressurised to be completely dry by a certain age. However, it should be made clear that this is not a substitute for careful and effective parenting. There are many reasons why a child might wet the bed, and pathological causes should also be explored. Note that a child under the age of 16 should never be treated alone: a parent or guardian should be present at all times.

It has been suggested that bedwetting children should avoid apples and apple juice, and foods with a malic acid content. In food products, the latter is shown as E296 and is also present in pears and some sweeteners. The reasoning and effectiveness behind this is largely anecdotal, but a build-up of malate in certain cells causes an imbalance of fluid movement. Avoiding these things does, however, seem to help, and the foods can be reintroduced gradually at a later stage. In these circumstances, a broad perspective and a very positive and supportive approach are needed from both the parent and the therapist.

CHAPTER 11

Diaphragm and Respiratory System

The diaphragm procedure is one that is most commonly associated with asthma, but nevertheless can be used for a whole host of other presentations, many of which are not necessarily connected with respiration. The diaphragm is traditionally considered to be a muscle sitting up underneath the ribcage, with some attachments further down on the dorsal spine, and stabilised by the quadratus lumborum. This traditional view is fine but doesn't give the whole picture. The diaphragm muscle is actually in fascial continuity with the transversus abdominis (TA) fascia and, overlying the deep fascia of the viscera, the parietal peritoneum. Looping back on itself, it creates a continual structure that reaches as far down as the pelvic floor.

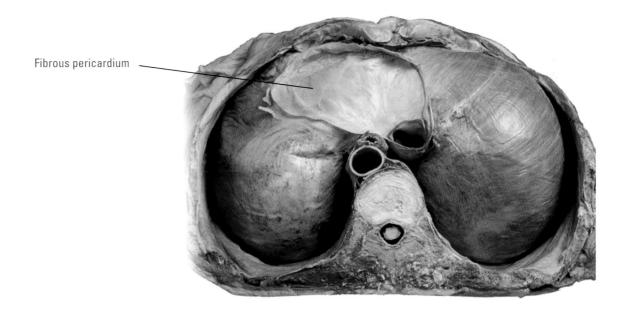

Fibrous pericardium

On top of the diaphragm is the heart. Usually represented as sitting on top of the diaphragm, the fibrous pericardium containing the heart is again a bag of fascia that is in continuity with the diaphragm and therefore an integral part of it. I was recently informed that in the UK, the pericardium is generally not repaired as part of a heart operation. It is hard to imagine what impact this might have on heart surgery patients in their recovery. It stands to reason, however, that if the importance of the fascial continuity is not established in the mind of the surgeon, then making changes to it isn't going to seem that important. We need to remember that surgery is still in its infancy, and procedures like heart surgery have only been successful for a very short space of time. I'm sure we still have a lot to learn.

With the heart so strongly attached to the diaphragm, it is potentially subject to diaphragmatic imbalances, and the procedure should be considered when heart conditions are present. Similarly the liver is held in place by a tendinous attachment to the diaphragm. As we breathe in and out, these attached organs are massaged and moved by this action, which takes place some twenty thousand times a day. Hence any move or procedure we make which might affect the diaphragm might reasonably also be expected to affect these organs as well.

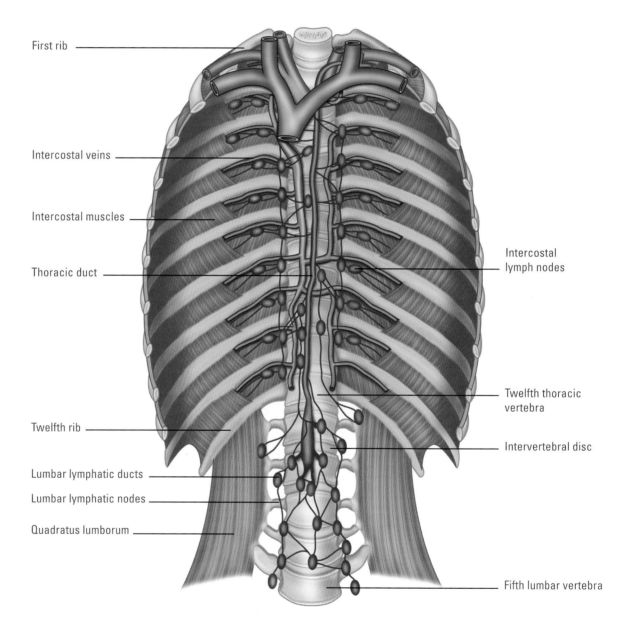

First rib

Intercostal veins

Intercostal muscles

Thoracic duct

Intercostal lymph nodes

Twelfth thoracic vertebra

Twelfth rib

Intervertebral disc

Lumbar lymphatic ducts

Lumbar lymphatic nodes

Quadratus lumborum

Fifth lumbar vertebra

Lymphatic drainage of the thoracic cavity.

Asthma is the most common respiratory condition, with nearly five million people in the UK having been diagnosed. However, any slight shortness of breath can sometimes be diagnosed as asthma with all the associated long-term pharmaceutical 'solutions'. In a vast number of cases, Bowen treatment has eliminated asthmatic symptoms in people diagnosed as asthmatic; in others, the respiratory function has increased, and better management of the asthmatic condition has resulted. The treatment using the diaphragm is of course also indicated for any respiratory presentation, including emphysema, pneumoconiosis, chronic obstructive pulmonary disease (COPD) and any situation where the drawing of breath is laboured, painful or compromised.

The simple element of muscular function is very rarely considered. Breath is the very essence of life and drives all the other functions of the body. We can't do without breathing, but we can do it badly for a long time. Poor or dysfunctional breathing in turn leads to a whole host of other problems, including poor digestion and bowel function, decreased ability to control pain, poor posture, stress, depression, migraine, poor sleep patterns, lack of concentration and so on. The diaphragm is also strongly indicated in lymphatic function. The whole act of breathing in and out creates a lymphatic movement, and poor breathing and posture will also contribute significantly to lymphatic congestion. In addition, there is a concentration of lymph nodes through the dorsal thoracic spine.

DIAPHRAGM AND BIOMECHANICAL FUNCTION

Whilst it is natural to associate the diaphragm with breathing and respiratory function, there is a whole host of other elements that need to be considered. The linking of breath with the restoration of normal function around the body is one area. In any chronic pain situation, we are likely to find people who are not breathing effectively or fully. This has the potential to create a downward spiral in terms of pain management, and will also restrict the ability of the body to repair and heal itself. In addition, if we are to see the diaphragm as a continuous structure, blended in with the fibres of the transversus abdominis, we also need to understand the functional and postural relationships that will be associated with this.

The pulling forwards and over-tensioning of the abdominal muscles will naturally restrict and contract the diaphragm, bringing the body into flexion. The diaphragm is in effect the upper part of a large bag, containing all the viscera and organs. This bag is called the parietal peritoneum and is encased at the top by the diaphragm, and around the midsection by the transversus abdominis; the bottom of the bag sits on the fibres of the pelvic floor.

As well as the massaging effect of the diaphragm on the organs already mentioned, there is also a functional element. If the pelvis is tilted one way or the other, this in turn has a potential effect on all the fibres associated with it, including the diaphragm. The upper body will also be compensating around the diaphragm, and if the ability of the body to breathe is being compromised, then the accessory muscles of respiration will start to play a larger role. Watch somebody with breathing difficulties and observe how their neck and shoulders behave when they are trying to draw a deep breath.

This behaviour also migrates into a mental approach. If you stand with your shoulders hunched, your head drooped and your arms folded, then the words "I feel happy and positive" are hardly likely to feel appropriate to your posture. Similarly, standing upright and pushing the chest out will enable most of us to be able to breathe better and feel more physically and mentally alert. The diaphragm is therefore a very useful adjunct to working with chronic pain as well as disease, even if respiratory problems are not a primary presentation. Helping someone to breathe more efficiently will always help them feel better.

MILK AND DAIRY

A key recommendation for clients with respiratory illness is to avoid dairy products, milk in particular. As a foodstuff, milk should be regarded as more of a luxury item than the staple it is considered to be in today's Western diet. Cow's milk is ultimately a food staple designed for baby cows, and, whilst there is a lot of evidence to suggest that raw milk has some benefits, the pasteurisation and homogenisation of milk creates a product that will not sustain a baby cow and takes away most of what could be deemed beneficial to the human digestive system.

Having mucus- and acid-forming properties, milk as a food staple, as well as the long and misleading idea of it being a great source of calcium, has seen it pervading all areas of food manufacturing. The mucus element is a potential issue for respiratory conditions, quite apart from the lactose intolerance that is prevalent in most humans. Milk should therefore be avoided, as should other triggers such as pollen, dust and the propellants from aerosol sprays.

Often seen in people suffering from asthma are skin conditions such as eczema. It is a positive indication of the respiratory problem being linked to an intestinal/stomach imbalance. In many cases this is what is causing both problems, and referral to a good nutritional practitioner could be very beneficial.

BABY COLIC

Anyone who has witnessed the sight (and sound) of a baby suffering from colic will attest to the level of distress that is experienced by both baby and parent. The causes of colic, as with asthma, are not entirely clear, and it is not inconceivable that the two are in someway linked. Similarly to asthma, there is little or no consideration of the diaphragm in the conventional treatment of colic, and many babies just have to 'grow out of it'.

As well as being very underdeveloped, the diaphragm in an infant has to work very hard. A baby will have a very fast heart rate and correspondingly high rate of respiration. A possible explanation of the pain of colic suggests some kind of knot or congestion around the underside of the diaphragm, which an immature respiratory system is unable to voluntarily cough up. The moves for colic are similar to a manually induced cough, and it is very common for a baby to vomit soon after. When this happens, the emission is often foul smelling and can also be accompanied by similar bowel movements. Unpleasant for all, but sweet relief from the pain and sleepless nights of a colicky baby.

CHEST PAINS

There are many circumstances in which someone might present with pains in their chest, the most obvious one being a heart attack. If there is any suggestion, or even the slightest chance, that this is the case, an ambulance must be called. However, it might be that someone is suffering either from a severe case of indigestion (a problem that has seen many people rushed to hospital with suspected heart attacks), or from inflammatory conditions of the costal area. In the case of indigestion, the standard diaphragm procedure should be fairly effective, but for more persistent problems, a remarkable effect can be achieved by slightly changing the Page Three moves we do after the diaphragm procedure.

The same will apply to spinal deformities such as scoliosis, kyphosis and lordosis. The idea is to create a spinal reference for the diaphragmatic work, rather than emphasising the whole upper body. It may sound strange, but we have witnessed some remarkable changes in spinal structures over the years, and the procedure is highly recommended where such types of problem exist.

EMERGENCIES

The diaphragm moves can be extremely effective in the case of an asthma attack. There are some 500 deaths and over 70,000 emergency hospital admissions a year in the UK from asthma, and yet there is no established first-aid principle in use.

This move is quite literally a life-saver, and there are many examples and stories of Bowen therapists using this in acute situations where the outcome might otherwise have been very serious. The move should always be done with the client standing and is not a substitute for emergency treatment. In the case of an acute asthma attack, an ambulance must always be called; the emergency move is simply given to slow down the process while waiting for the emergency services to arrive.

THE BOWEN ASTHMA EMERGENCY MOVE

When either an adult or a child has an asthma attack, their chest will become tighter and tighter. In a small child or baby, the stomach will also appear to collapse inwards. The asthma emergency move can release the diaphragm tension, and will allow the person to breathe more easily. If they have pain in the centre of their chest, this will usually go away immediately, with the diaphragm releasing over the next few minutes. In minor cases, the tension may take several minutes to release, but will work in a very similar manner to the bronchodilator, often called the 'puffer', and will last much longer. It is a simple move, easily done by the victim or a parent, and has saved lives on several notable occasions.

Locate the xiphoid process below the sternum (breast bone). Using a thumb or finger, find a point about an inch below this. Take up the skin slack, apply gentle pressure, and pull the thumb/finger down reasonably quickly. Care should be taken not to use too much pressure. Those affected during exercise or sport can use this move about 15 minutes prior to commencing the activity, and at any time they feel any tightness. It can be safely used, albeit gently, on small children and babies, and can help with persistent coughing.

Many asthma sufferers now use this release move in preference to their 'puffer'; in a large number of cases, the need for the 'puffer' nearly been eliminated. This move can be demonstrated to an adult, child or parent, and can be repeated as often as needed. Advise the subject to do it at least twice a day for the first week: this will ensure that they not only learn how to use it, but also remember to use it when necessary, rather than resorting to using the 'puffer' first.

Because the diaphragm will tighten in a similar way when someone has either a panic attack or an anxiety attack, the move can be successfully used to release tension and calm the person down. Copies of the release move can be downloaded from the Internet (see http://www.bowen-for-asthma.com or http://www.relieve-childhood-asthma.com).

BREAKDOWN

The diaphragm is innervated by the phrenic nerve, which emerges from the neck at C3–C5 and runs down in front of the scalenus. It provides motor innervations to the diaphragm and is responsible for the act of breathing. It also provides sensation for a lot of other areas around the chest, as well as the upper abdomen, the liver and the gall bladder. This means that problems coming from the heart (such as angina), from the liver (such as an abscess or growth) or from the chest (such as a fractured rib), all areas served by the phrenic nerve, can often be referred into the shoulder, neck or arm.

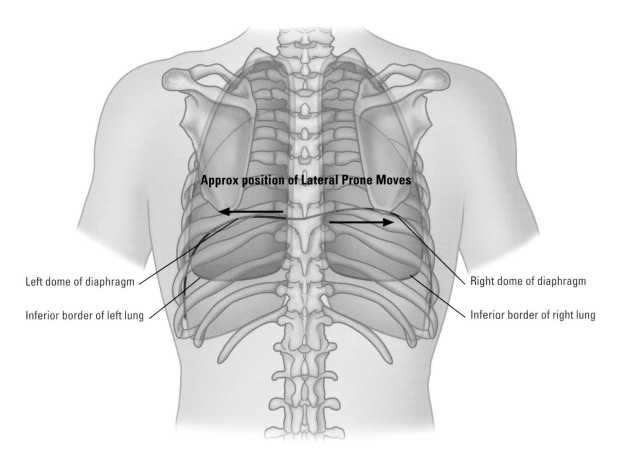

Here is yet another reminder that the initial moves of Pages One to Three are incredibly important, and demonstrates the effectiveness of Bowen in taking the whole body into account.

The diaphragm and respiratory procedure works by diverting energy which is focused on the primary curve of the mid-thoracic area, into the junction of the lung and diaphragm.

THE LEG LOCK EXPLAINED

When we lift the leg up and outwards, the entire trunk will move, slightly rotating under the pressure of our hand on the ankle. As we have already seen, the diaphragm is continuous with the muscles and tissues of the abdomen and trunk, and will therefore move and slightly rotate together with the rest of this area. At a certain point, the diaphragm will not be moving; it is this point, at which a change in the movement is felt, that we are looking for. It can be quite hard to locate, but by a combination of observation and palpation we can generally locate the right spot. If we can't see or feel this area, then making the move on a line slightly above where the upper stoppers start will do just as well.

The move aims to work the junction of the diaphragm where it meets the lung, creating a junctional relationship and where clear movement is essential for effective respiratory function. In the chest area, the fascia that surrounds the ribs and the area into the abdomen is not layered in straight lines, but is oriented diagonally, in effect creating a line from the shoulder to the opposite hip. By working with this line of energetic strain, we allow a big surge of stored kinetic energy to be released via the abdominal muscle and fascia. The underside of the ribs is where the transversus abdominis connects up to the diaphragm. Just like a junction where two raging rivers meet, the differentiated directions of the two muscles create a very energetic meeting point.

The last move, down from the xiphoid, drops the diaphragm and creates a balance between the thoracic and abdominal areas. The abdominal area is thus dealt with, as are the relationships already discussed.

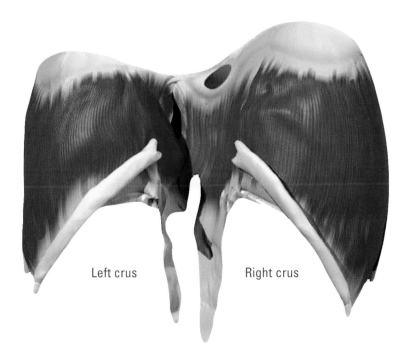

Left crus   Right crus

On the front, the moves set up a kind of opposition effect. Whereas when the client was prone we moved across the right side first, when the client is supine, we work across the left side first.

There is also a need for the diaphragm to be stabilised. This is facilitated by two long arms called 'crus', which reach down to the front part of the longitudinal ligament of the lumbar spine and blend in around L1 to L3. The crus also have a strong fascial relationship with the psoas major and are continuous with this muscle before blending into the longitudinal ligament.

In a kind of trapeze act, other muscles help to stabilise the diaphragm, coming up from the pelvis in the shape of the quadratus lumborum (QL). The QL is a large, flat muscle of the posterior abdominal wall, and lies deep to the erector spinae and psoas major. It is a difficult area to palpate, but if done carefully, and in the right position, there are some very effective Bowen moves which achieve great results for respiratory conditions as well as for problems associated with a lifted pelvis. The QL references to the twelfth rib, and through the rib helping to hold the QL down, the muscle works by assisting stabilisation of the lower attachments of the diaphragm, allowing it to contract more effectively. So – a back pain might even take the breath away? Stabilising and releasing moves for the QL will help to restore a functioning posture, in turn allowing easier and clearer respiration.

Additionally, the system needs to have access to all the oxygenated blood supply it can get. Chronic pain, lack of sleep, infection and so forth will all have an impact both on the breathing and on the way in which the body is held. It is worth thinking about working the diaphragm, as well as other areas, even when it is not that obvious.

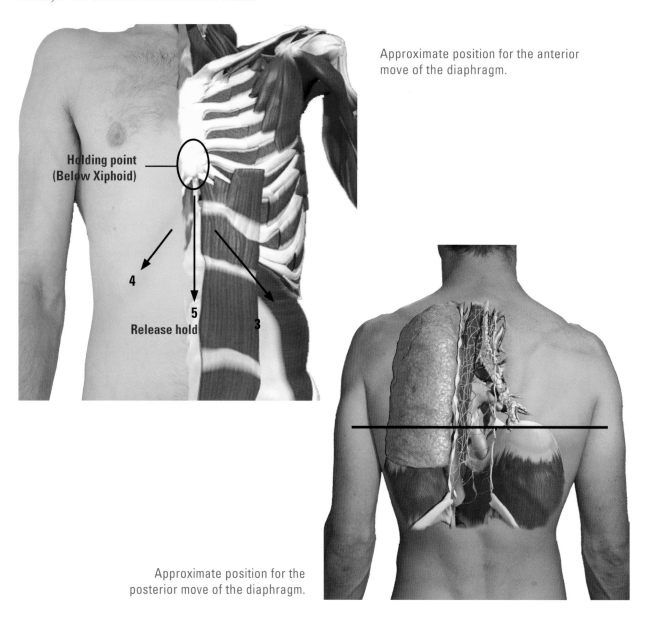

Approximate position for the anterior move of the diaphragm.

Holding point
(Below Xiphoid)

4

5
Release hold

3

Approximate position for the posterior move of the diaphragm.

CHAPTER 12

Elbow

The elbow procedure is quite complex, made up of both moves and holding points; it encompasses moves from the elbow down to and including the wrist. Unlike most other procedures, the elbow one is fairly localised, and there are not likely to be many presentations other than elbow and wrist that will be affected by this procedure. However, there are several other areas to consider in addition to the elbow when treating elbow, forearm and wrist problems. This is particularly the case with a so-called repetitive strain injury (RSI). Many people presenting with arm pain, tennis elbow and especially RSI need to be questioned about any history of neck pain or injury, and this area should be considered in the treatment.

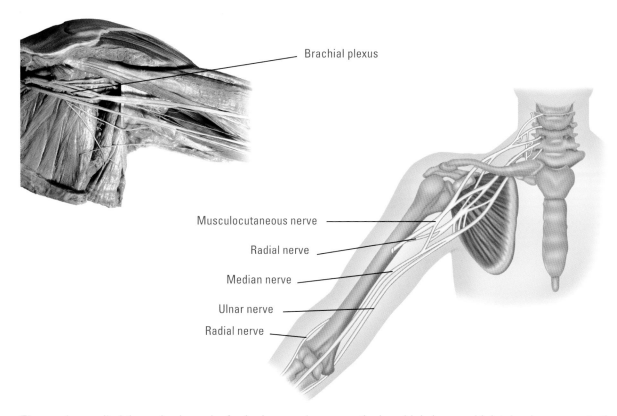

Brachial plexus

Musculocutaneous nerve

Radial nerve

Median nerve

Ulnar nerve

Radial nerve

The arm is supplied through a branch of spinal nerves known as the brachial plexus, which takes in, amongst others, the median, ulnar and radial nerves.

The position of the head and neck in relation to the rest of the upper body, and even the lower back, is going to have an effect on nerve supply to the arms. A head held forwards, a tilted pelvis or a head compensating for an upper thoracic restriction or pain will all have the potential for presenting symptoms of pain in the arms and hands. A classic posture occurs during pregnancy, where many women present with carpal tunnel syndrome or tendinous pains in their forearms. I believe that this is as much to do with the biomechanics of pregnancy as it is anything else, and again the position of the pelvis, and the subsequent compensations that need to take place in the shoulders, will be significantly involved.

The ability of the client to laterally flex the neck (side bending) is an important one when assessing any form of arm and shoulder problem. Any restriction here suggests a potential 'bulking-up' of fascial tissue and might therefore be the starting point of treatment. The emphasis is, once again, on Pages Two and Three, covering areas that need to be worked on before the elbow or arm is addressed. The jaw and temporomandibular joint is another area which may be involved in nerve supply to the arms and should also be considered.

The elbow area can, of course, also be damaged or painful with no other mitigating factors, and localised or isolated injury or inflammation is not uncommon. The term 'tennis elbow' refers to lateral epicondylitis – inflammation of the lateral epicondyle (funny bone). The repetitive movements of pronating and supinating the hand are exaggerated when under pressure. The action of hitting a tennis ball is typical of the kind of action that would create this kind of pain. Another example would be using a screwdriver to press down on a screw, with the arm being twisted at the same time.

'Golfer's elbow', or medial epicondylitis, similarly refers to the opposing action when contacting a golf ball. Both this and tennis elbow would be addressed in the same way as far as Bowen is concerned, using the elbow procedure after Pages Two and Three have been performed. With the golf swing, there is also the potential to cause a jarring injury to the joint, and repetitive injuries are

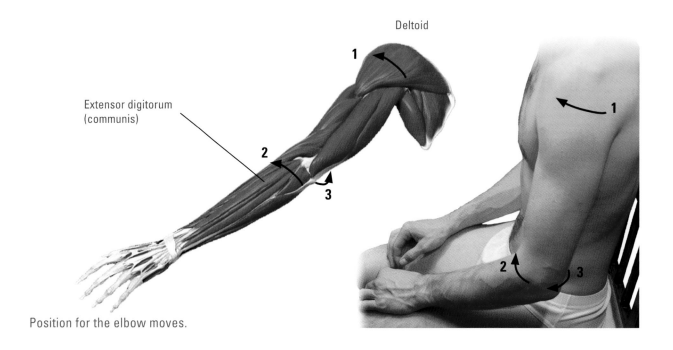

Position for the elbow moves.

common. A big help, in relation to treating many sporting injuries, is to recommend the services of a professional coach. Many, if not most, amateur golfers will be self-taught, mid-handicap, weekend players. A few sessions with someone addressing their swing will almost certainly help to eliminate the kind of damaging patterns that create injury and strain. The same can be said for most sports.

The moves of the elbow are reasonably location specific, and, whilst there is a degree of margin for error, there is plenty of scope for adding more moves and developing the way that the procedure is put together. Once learned, the procedure itself takes a few seconds to perform. For the first move we look at the mid-deltoid, which attaches down onto the upper part of the humerus. The shoulder may well have already been addressed as part of the overall treatment of the arm, but the mid-deltoid is the missing link here. Again, I refer back to the clear and strong connection of the deltoid to the trapezius, which we have seen in the pictures of upper body dissections (see page 49).

The second move works across the extensor digitorum communis, a group of extensor muscles in the forearm which are referred to as 'communis' because they share the same bag of fascia. The middle finger can often be seen to flick slightly when this move is made. The object of this single move is to connect the forearm through the complex joint of the elbow and set up the next move from the back of the epicondyle.

The third move of the elbow has been the cause of much debate over the years, primarily in regard to the exact structures being addressed. For simplicity we can use the triceps tendon as a reference

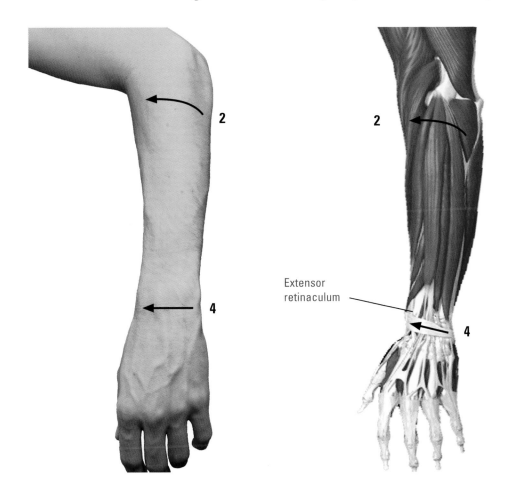

Extensor retinaculum

Elbow moves 2 and 4.

point, although it should be noted that working the biceps on the inside of the elbow can also prove useful. The concept of the hold is to create a short-term numbing effect through the elbow joint, and allow pain-free extension of the arm to take place. The pressure either side of the epicondyle is onto the median and ulnar nerves, whilst the thumb applies pressure to the radiohumeral joint, situated between the head of the radius and the end of the humerus. The pressures should be applied for around 10–15 seconds, or until any unusual sensations are felt in the fingers: these could be tingling, numbness or coldness, and will indicate that the hold should be released at once.

Immediately following the holding of the joint, the fourth move is performed to work the extensor retinaculum over the base of the wrist. In anatomy books this extensor seems to exist as a separate entity from the rest of the fascia of the arm. In fact, the retinaculum fibres found over many joints in the body are simply thickened areas of the fascial continuity. They appear as they do, once the rest of the fascia has been trimmed away and discarded. The function of these thick bands is to create a taping effect through which tendons can move and be held in place.

At this point in the wrist, the fascia also serves to keep a grip on the myriad bones of the joint, which get little in the way of natural movement under normal circumstances. The stretch and rotation of this joint is therefore a useful mobiliser for the forearm and wrist, and should be done under pressure, with the thumbs pointing up the arm. It is important that the wrist does not drop downwards during this figure-of-eight movement, as this would put pressure on the flexor retinaculum at the back of the wrist – something we are trying to avoid.

A short flick and downward pull through the wrist creates an opening of the three joints of the arm, but should be done gently and with due consideration for the normal range of movement of the arm. The 'snake' follows: this is aimed at realigning the three bones of the arm and is what all the rest of the moves have been leading to. The therapist should first 'rehearse' the movement a few times with the client, helping them to create the rotational-type movement which is needed to allow the arm to fully extend and rotate. The hand must be extended away at the start of this movement, and supinated at the end. Any attempt to begin the sharp movement with the hand turned inwards will create pressure on the joint and lead to the unpleasant possibility of a dislocation through the olecranon of the elbow.

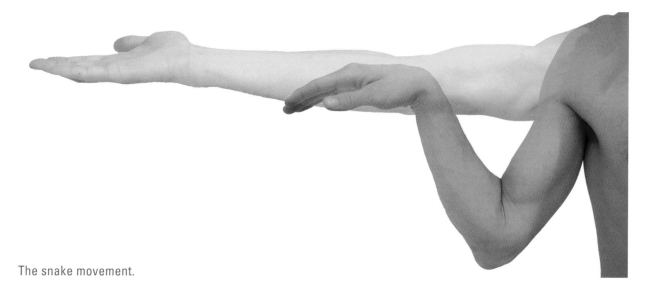

The snake movement.

The click that is often heard at this point is an indication that the move has been successful. If the problem really is tennis elbow, then this move should resolve the issue almost immediately, although care should be taken to avoid repeating the action that caused the original problem. Strengthening exercises would be advisable.

In days gone by, the adjustment of the elbow was performed by the therapist, who applied upward pressure under the elbow. The idea of the client performing the snake was in response to this adjustment being deemed a chiropractic manoeuvre, something which became outlawed in Australia with the advent of chiropractic registration. Even so, it remains a method of choice for some, particularly where the client is unable to naturally perform the rotational movement of the arm. The manoeuvre does, however, need to have been taught and should never be attempted by the therapist unless they have been trained to do it.

Carpal tunnel syndrome – defined as pressure on the median nerve through the flexor retinaculum, the thick fascial banding on the underside of the wrist – also needs to have the rest of the arm, the shoulder and the neck considered and possibly treated. The median nerve, being part of the brachial plexus, is vulnerable to pressure from both the neck and the shoulder. As we have already discussed, in cases where both wrists are experiencing symptoms of carpal tunnel syndrome, it is unlikely that the problem originates solely from the wrists. Teasing out of the anterior aspect of the forearm, along the line of the median nerve, has proved remarkably successful with carpal tunnel syndrome, and, naturally enough, is a much-preferred option to surgery. Even where surgery is scheduled, this procedure is vital in order to prevent the scarring that commonly follows.

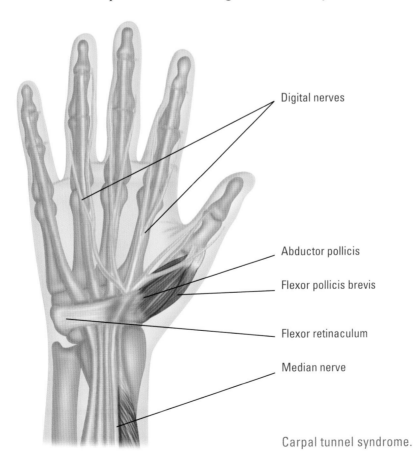

Digital nerves

Abductor pollicis

Flexor pollicis brevis

Flexor retinaculum

Median nerve

Carpal tunnel syndrome.

REPETITIVE STRAIN INJURY (RSI)

The subject of RSI is somewhat controversial. Many people working in offices, factories and supermarkets have made RSI-related compensation claims over the years, and have suffered severe problems and pains in their arms and hands, resulting in quite crippling disability in some cases. However, whilst many people will claim to have been injured as a result of using, for instance, a mouse and a keyboard, many more people who use these tools suffer no problems at all. It could therefore be suggested that if any given job gave you RSI, the majority of people doing said job would experience similar problems.

In the 1970s and 1980s many mineworkers using vibrational machinery for long periods found that, as a result, they suffered irreparable damage to their hands, a condition known as 'vibration white finger'. A cover-up by the Coal Board management at the time meant that many men continued to use machinery in a manner which would eventually permanently disable them – the nerves in their hands shaken, quite literally, to death.

The same cannot be said of using a keyboard. However, doing anything incorrectly, with a poor posture, at the wrong height and without the appropriate training and breaks, can end up giving someone problems. Add to this mix a previous neck, upper back or shoulder condition, even a habitual posture, and the result will be similar. Workplace conditions can therefore be seen to contribute to an RSI condition, whilst not exactly causing it.

The point here is that we cannot view RSI as a separate condition, but must instead look at the wider picture and aim to restore function to, and normal supply from, areas other than the hands and forearms. The moves across the extensors that have been taught to many have very little effect in terms of treating RSI or any wider problem, but might have the benefit of reassuring the client that the area of concern has been addressed.

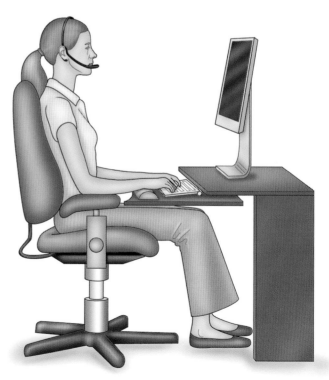

Ideal work posture to prevent potential RSI conditions?

CHAPTER 13

Hamstrings

The hamstring group is traditionally, although erroneously, thought of as a problem area in sportsmen and women. Tight or torn hamstrings are often the cause of long layoffs from competing, and particularly so in more severe cases. A hamstring strain is the most common sports-related lower limb injury, with a high risk of recurrence and lengthy recovery times (Dadebo et al. 2004, Hoskins and Pollard 2005, Gabbe et al. 2005). In professional sport this can represent an expensive period of treatment and even involve surgical intervention. Stretching, the usual approach to prevention and treatment of hamstring injuries, has been challenged in recent times; some reports suggest that stretching the hamstrings can actually increase the risk of injury, because of the desensitisation of the stretch reflex (Shyne and Dominguez 1982; Saal 1987; Murphy 1991; Gleim and McHugh 1997).

Short or tight hamstrings are also implicated in a host of other related problems in the knee, ankle and foot and in the lower back. The key thing to remember when considering the hamstrings is that this is essentially a pelvic muscle, joining onto a strong ligament to create a large amount of tension through the leg and into the sacrum. The long head of the biceps femoris joins with the semitendinosus to

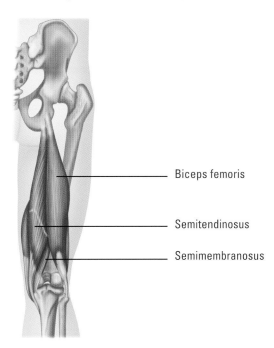

Biceps femoris

Semitendinosus

Semimembranosus

form a strong muscular attachment to the ischial tuberosity. However, far from this being the end of the story, this attachment serves as a reference point for the continuing journey of the hamstrings into the thickened cushion of fascia sitting in and around the sacrum and lower back.

The traditional attachment of the biceps femoris seems to be in two parts. The anterior aspect of it is indeed fixed quite firmly to the fascia of the ischial tuberosity. However, the posterior part is in direct continuity with the sacrotuberous ligament. This relationship appears at times to be similar to a synovial joint – smooth and movable – yet under extreme tensions and pressures from below and above. Even so, movement and absorption of force through the structure is well demonstrated. The sacrotuberous ligament then blends into the fascia of the sacrum, and becomes completely untraceable as it diverges and blends into the fascia of dozens of other structures in the area, in a multidirectional mass of darting fibres. The lateral part of the long dorsal sacroiliac ligament is also continuous with the fibres of the sacrotuberous ligament, and has fibres connected to the deep lamina of the thoracolumbar fascia, to the erector spinae and to the multifidus (Vleeming et al. 1996).

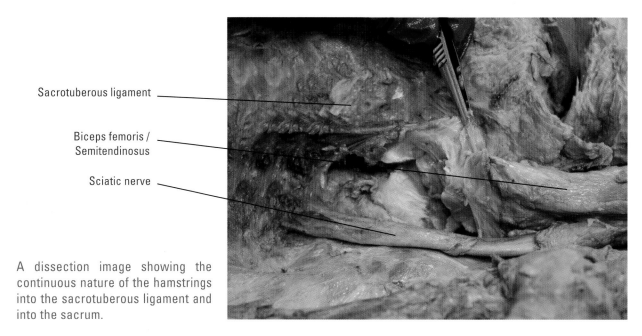

Sacrotuberous ligament

Biceps femoris / Semitendinosus

Sciatic nerve

A dissection image showing the continuous nature of the hamstrings into the sacrotuberous ligament and into the sacrum.

Traditionally referred to as the thoracolumbar fascia, this multilayered material acts as a kind of muscular fuse box for the whole body, mediating signals through it to a network of fascial connections. It is perhaps only a small exaggeration to suggest that virtually every muscle in the body is connected directly or indirectly to the fascia around the sacrum. The concept of strains being sent through the body in lines of tension, such as proposed in Tom Myer's Anatomy Trains theory, explains the concept of structural continuity very well. However, when the complexity of the sacral fascia is examined, we can see that the strain is not going to be transmitted along predetermined lines, but will instead transmit through wherever the pressure is placed, or when movement creates demand to initiate function. To demonstrate this concept, consider the pile of hands in the picture.

Somewhere in there is a hand at the bottom of the pile, under considerable pressure from all the others. If this hand moves, even slightly, every other hand can feel that movement. If the hand on top pulls in a different direction to the hand at the bottom, the hands in the middle will feel this contrary pull. They in turn can also push or pull to create movement extending into every other hand in the pile.

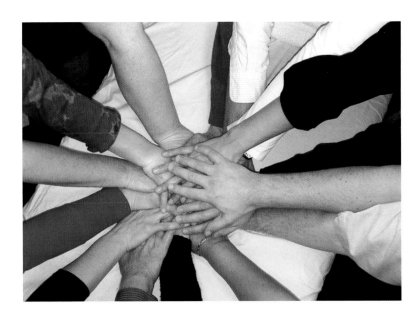

Each hand will be able to feel the movement of every other hand and respond accordingly.

However, the fascia in the sacral area is not layered in the simple way that the hands are, but instead blend into each other, creating indistinguishable pushes and pulls throughout the area. Simply put, we can see that a shortening or tightening of the hamstrings has the potential to create strains throughout the whole body, from the soles of the feet to the top of the head, either along the same side of the body or even crossing over to the opposite side as a more likely transference of strain.

We must therefore view the hamstrings as being a major tensional component of the whole of the back, to be taken into account when making assessments of the knees, ankles, thoracic spine and in particular the pelvis. The nature of the hamstrings being wrapped in the white fascial banding around the leg means that the iliotibial band will also be involved and affected by hamstring shortening or injury.

From a muscular perspective, the hamstring and lower leg grouping can be seen as a co-operative network, similar to the grip used by trapeze artists, with the gastrocnemius and soleus working in co-operation with the hamstrings to create a perfect tensional relationship. When you stand upright, the grouping kicks in, and the tension is extended from the bottom of the feet all the way up the back and into the neck. The smallest bit of flexion through the knees releases this tension.

In the sporting arena, tight hamstrings will inevitably lead to injury, but not always to the hamstrings themselves. The beauty of this procedure is that the effects of the moves continue for some time after the treatment is finished. A research programme undertaken by Michelle Marr and colleagues at the European College of Bowen Studies (ECBS) and Coventry University, studying the effects of Bowen on hamstring flexibility, found that not only did the flexibility increase immediately post-treatment, but also this increase was maintained and even improved over the following seven days (Marr et al. 2011). In a passive treatment this is virtually unheard of and raises many questions as to what is happening in fascial tissue during the treatment, but also especially in the hours and even days afterwards.

It seems inescapable, however, that there is an unwinding effect through the tissues which, although seen immediately in many cases, continues long after the therapist has finished the treatment. This effect is not unusual in Bowen, with many clients leaving the treatment room in exactly the same condition as when they arrived. Whilst this can sometimes be a cause of concern for sports therapists or other remedial bodyworkers, the Bowen therapist should never be concerned. It is an important point to remember when confronted with so-called 'advanced Bowen' in which lots of work is performed. Let the body do the work!

HAMSTRINGS AS STABILISERS

A recent case history obliterated the myth that the more flexible the hamstrings the better. A 39-year-old teacher presented with virtually constant lower-back pain on normal movement. He had no sharp pains or particularly limited ranges of movement, but after a couple of hours of standing and normal moving around, he was in constant discomfort across the top of the ilium. Various treatments had been tried, and whilst there had been some limited relief, the pain always returned. The usual suspects had been eliminated, and X-rays and scans showed nothing in the way of significant wear or damage. What intrigued me was his reporting that he felt almost total relief when lying on his back with his legs bent. What was it about this position that took the strain off the back?

The teacher reported that he was very flexible and had been a gymnast as a young man. On inspection he was able to bend very easily, and rest the palms of his hands on the floor. When the strength of his flexion was tested while he was lying face down, he was unable to push against my hand to any degree at all. It was a light-bulb moment when my feelings and ideas on connective tissue and integrative medicine came together. Simply put, the teacher's hamstrings were too flexible and were not giving him enough support in the lower half of his body.

This meant that all the work of keeping his pelvis in place fell to the muscles of the lower back. A couple of hours into a day and they really began to feel the strain. Lying down makes the floor the stabiliser and takes the strain off the back. The analogy here is to that of a hammock, with the mat area being the pelvis and the strings at either end being the spinal muscles and the hamstrings. These fibres, although appearing to have an identity at either end of the hammock, are in fact completely integrated into the structure. Without an effectual tensional relationship, the mat of the hammock is going to be very unstable and effectively unusable. Therefore, not only will the hamstring procedure increase flexibility in the hamstrings, it seems it can also decrease flexibility and strengthen the muscle where needed. After the simple moves on the hamstrings, his strength increased and the back pain decreased dramatically.

It is not the first time this situation has been witnessed. In the research programme that addressed the flexibility of the hamstrings using Bowen (Marr et al. 2011), we also saw a very mobile client attain a reduced range of movement and therefore more stability. In the battle between stability and flexibility, it is normally stability that wins. We become immobile and stiff very easily. Yet there are occasions when excessive mobility will lead to instability as in the case of the teacher. It appears that Bowen can sort this either way.

All this seems to suggest that there is some kind of innate mechanism whereby connective tissue will return to a default state if given the correct stimulus – a principle which is plausible if we study the ability of fascia to contract and expand independently of muscle tissue. Lots more future study and research in this area will no doubt give us a better idea of what is really happening, but for now we just have to work with the results.

PREVENTION IS BETTER THAN CURE

Hamstring injuries in sports can be difficult to resolve, but the best position to be in is the one in which the athlete doesn't get injured in the first place. This holds true within all areas of sport, yet is not given the consideration it deserves. A sportsperson at the peak of their physical fitness should not be in such a position that they are constantly picking up injuries. The whole field of sports injury plays into the idea that sport in general is something that is likely to result in injury. Whilst any type of contact sport is going to knock the body about, there is no real reason why an active, fit person should be plagued by constant setbacks. The clue is in the fact that the majority of sporting injuries are repeat presentations of old injuries.

This leads us to two suppositions. Firstly, the original injury may not have been completely rehabilitated or dealt with properly, or perhaps it stemmed from somewhere other than the site of the presentation. Secondly, it might be that the weakness of the original injury has continued to create compensations and strains, leading to a build-up of tension and a repeat of the injury.

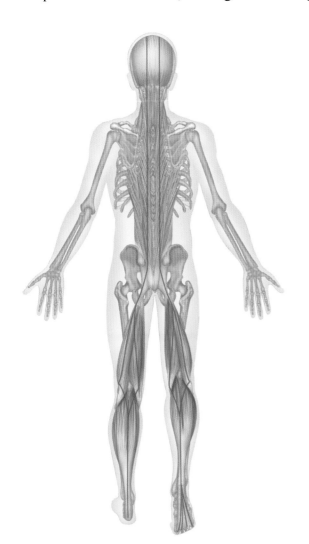

The superficial back line model in Anatomy Trains.

This is the nature of injury, however. Tension creates the potential for injury in much the same way as a tight piece of plastic tears or becomes damaged more easily than a relaxed one. Once damage occurs, any repair that is attempted under tension will always be slower and more difficult to achieve, with the result that a reoccurrence of the injury is more likely.

The hamstring procedure is therefore an ideal preventative tool for many types of lower limb, back and abdominal injury. Many sportsmen and women find that, with regular treatments, the incidence of injury is significantly decreased. Sports therapists who use preventative Bowen treatments report a big reduction in the number of hamstring strains and pulls.

SCIATIC NERVE

The sciatic nerve is made up of the tibial and common peroneal nerves. These two nerves sit together in a thick band that runs down the back of the leg and (in most people) in between the hamstrings. The band separates near the knee to become the two nerves mentioned. It is a big, thick bundle and subject to lots of external pressures and biomechanical influences; there are many variations of how and where it sits.

A common presentation is what people refer to as 'sciatica', which, if taken literally, means an inflammation of the sciatic nerve. In most cases, however, what they are experiencing is pain radiating down the leg, and this is more often than not caused by pressure on the nerve rather than inflammation or damage to it. Given the nerve's location, the hamstring procedure would be a good place to start with sciatic-type pain. Another, even simpler, approach with a male subject is to check to see if he carries his wallet in his back pocket. If so, suggest that he remove it and keep it elsewhere!

BENDING THE KNEE

The knee is bent at a right angle during the prone part of the procedure for one simple reason: to prevent contraction of the hamstrings, which the client would be able to do if the knee were bent at an angle greater than 90 degrees. Because you will be putting a reasonable amount of pressure on this area, a contraction would potentially be quite painful. By putting the knee into flexion, the muscle grouping is effectively switched off (similar to switching off the power supply to an electrical appliance), and work can safely be done in this area.

When the jar is made to the metatarsal heads of the foot, most of the work of the hamstring procedure has been accomplished. You will often see a reflex all the way through to the head and neck, more often on the opposite side to the one you are working. This jar creates vibrational movement throughout the line of the calf and hamstring and into the back. Recent studies using biofeedback machines have suggested that the jar gives resonant readings even as far as the fingers of each hand.

The jar to the metatarsal ball of the foot needs to be a firm one if it is going to have the effect we are looking for. It is not simply symbolic but instead powerful enough to create a distinct and sharp pull through the back of the leg and into the sacrum. A gentle tap at this point just isn't going to cut the ice.

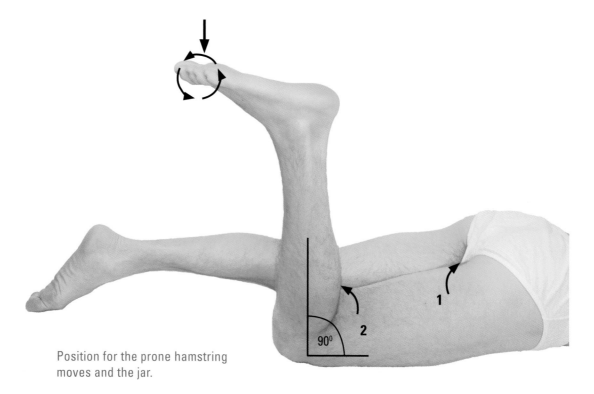

Position for the prone hamstring moves and the jar.

The five-minute break indicated in the notes is to allow the client time to rest and for the jarred nerve endings to settle. You have made quite a big move here, and the body needs a chance to work out what has been relaxed and what has been contracted. It doesn't matter whether you leave them to rest prone, or whether you turn them over. Hit the lat and then leave them for the five minutes.

The moves on the back of the leg performed when the client is supine are more for relaxing the leg and the calf. The idea is to try to separate the muscles of the hamstring group, namely the biceps femoris, semitendinosus and semimembranosus. Do not come too far up the leg for the first move, as these three muscles come together at a certain point, although this is rarely accurately illustrated. As we have already moved over this with our elbow, the aim is to find a point at which they can be separated.

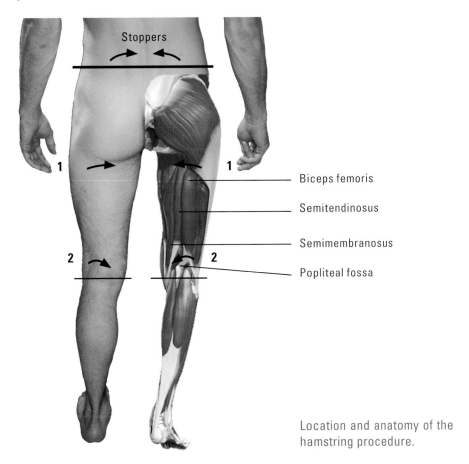

Biceps femoris

Semitendinosus

Semimembranosus

Popliteal fossa

Location and anatomy of the hamstring procedure.

KNEE AND HAMSTRING PROCEDURES COMBINED

If performing the knee and hamstring procedures together, complete the hamstrings as described, all the way to the back of the knee on both sides. The three moves on the calf muscles are not needed, as the knee procedure will take care of this area. A break can be taken before coming back and starting the knee procedure, the first move still being the HTL.

The moves of the hamstring procedure are made mainly to join up the calf with the continuous line of the hamstrings, and to create an opening and relaxation. The knee moves are more numerous and fine, to help the drainage of the knee. The hamstring calf moves do not need to be performed in addition to the knee drainage moves. It's not really a problem if they are, it's just unnecessary time being taken up.

CHAPTER 14

Kidney

The kidney is the master chemist of the body. Sitting quietly nestled under the ribcage, it does the job of cleaning the junk that we insist on piling into our systems. If we examine the label of a packet of food and read that there are any number of interfered-with ingredients, then it is the kidneys that will have to handle most of the fall out. Caffeine, alcohol, salt and sugar are also elements which the kidney might have to deal with on a regular basis. Over 200 litres (or 350 pints) of water a day pass through the kidneys, in an endless recycling and cleansing of the blood, which means that we need to keep our intake of fluids regular if the kidneys are not to be stressed. There is such a thing as taking in too much water, though, and as with all things there is a balance to be maintained.

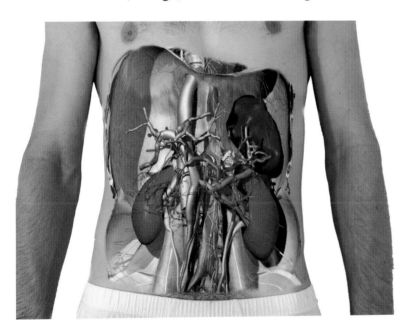

Location of the kidneys from the front.

With every breath we take, we lose water, and the body can lose naturally up to two litres of water a day, with very little energy expenditure. Most of this is made up by the food and drink that we consume, but the consumption of small, regular sips of water is recommended. For those sweating profusely for extended periods, the use of sports drinks as a hydrator is useful, as they contain salts, sugars and minerals, but tend to be over-sweet, ironically making the kidneys work harder and restricting the hydrating effect.

The kidneys are also quite involved in chemical adjustments in the body, adjusting the level of salts and minerals needed at any point in time. These organs also adjust the temperature of the body, as well as being part of the systems that address blood pressure.

Perched atop each kidney is a triangle-shaped adrenal gland, which produces steroid hormones. The gland has several functions, including maintaining normal blood pressure by balancing sodium, potassium and fluid levels. The adrenal cortex also makes small amounts of sex hormones, namely testosterone and oestrogen.

In addition, the glucocorticoids cortisol and corticosterone regulate blood pressure, support normal muscle function, promote protein breakdown, distribute body fat and increase blood sugar as needed. These hormones are mostly noted for their anti-inflammatory properties, hence the popularity of artificial cortisone as a medication. DHEA, or dehydroepiandrosterone, is another steroid hormone produced by the adrenals. Don't worry, you don't have to learn this – it is just interesting! The functions of this hormone are still rather unclear, but it appears to affect your heart, body weight, nervous system, immunity and bones as well as other systems.

Then there is our favourite word – stress! The inside of the adrenal gland is derived from the same type of tissue as the cells of the sympathetic ganglion. The steroid hormones from this inner part, namely epinephrine (also called adrenalin) and norepinephrine, are also controlled by the sympathetic nervous system during fear or stress. The body reacts to these hormones with the fight-or-flight response already discussed: a pounding heart, dilated pupils and raised blood pressure. The kidneys not only have to respond in times of stress, but also have to then perform the mopping-up process after the response has been felt by the rest of the system. Coming down from a highly stressed situation can take several days, often resulting in a 'crash' scenario as witnessed by rescue workers at the Twin Towers in New York after the 9/11 attacks in 2001.

Besides the chemistry of the kidneys and the adrenal system, there is also quite an emotional link which ties in with all of this – anger, frustration and being generally p***ed off! Feelings linked to long-term anger are likely to stress the kidneys, as well as of course disturbing the mental and emotional equilibrium of the client. Add to this mix the likelihood of destructive behaviour in highly stressed individuals, together with surrounding food, alcohol and drug use, and it is the kidneys which will take a beating.

The kidneys are entirely surrounded by two cushioning and protective layers of adipose, or superficial fascia, called the perirenal fat, which is part of the renal capsule. In addition to acting as protection, this fatty layer might also be involved in hormonal distribution. Pain in the kidney area, urinary tract infections and gout might all indicate kidney problems.

The kidneys also play an important role in lymphatic drainage and general function, as well as in the health of the immune system, and should be thought of as general regulators for overall healthy balance. For the most part, this balance goes unnoticed, but kidney problems are probably some of the most debilitating illnesses we can have. Jews even have a prayer, recited after using the toilet, called Asher Yatzar, which gives thanks for good health and the ability to excrete.

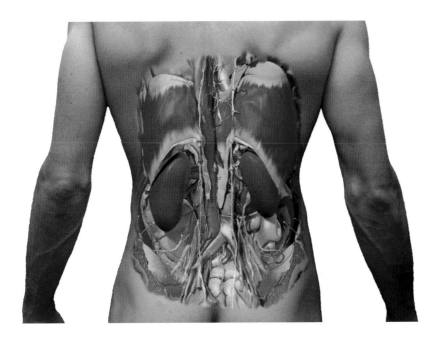

Kidney procedure.

APPLICATION

The move in this instance is made over the worst or most affected kidney, if it can be established. We can do this by firstly asking the client whether they are aware of a weakness in either kidney or even if there is pain in this region on either side. The second way we can determine the worst kidney is to look for any heat or difference in temperature. If one side is hot or warmer than normal body temperature, then, for this purpose, it is the indicated side. If neither side is tender, warm or otherwise indicated, we start with the moves on the right side. This is because apparently the right kidney is the one that tends to break down first if failure is going to happen.

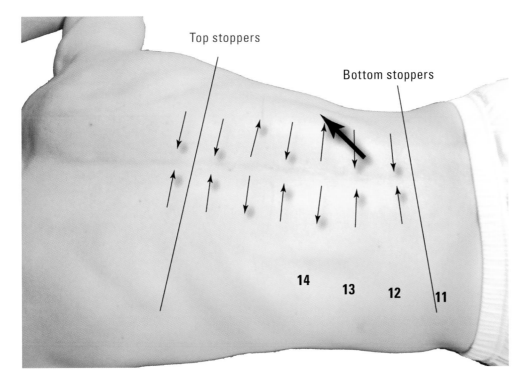

Kidney procedure with relevant stoppers.

The idea of the move is to take the energetic release achieved from performing moves 11–14 of Page Two and send this towards the affected kidney. It is a very powerful move and one which has had some interesting effects on clients over the years! The client's leg, raised on the same side that the therapist is standing, together with the client's head turned to the same side, creates a space into the renal cavity and directs the location and direction of the move.

BEETROOT

The use of beetroot as a cleanser for the liver and kidneys is widespread and has a very long history. It has even been considered to be an aphrodisiac since Roman times owing to its high levels of boron, which plays an important role in sex hormones. Beetroot provides a good source of anthocyanidins, a natural antioxidant that contributes to its deep-red colour, and is also particularly rich in vitamin C, calcium, phosphorus and iron. It has traditionally been used as a blood-building food for thousands of years.

Beetroot is rich in the nutrient betaine. Betaine supplements, manufactured as a by-product of sugar beet processing, are prescribed for lowering potentially toxic levels of homocysteine (Hcy). High levels of Hcy can be harmful to blood vessels, thus contributing to the development of heart disease, stroke and peripheral vascular disease. Beetroot is best taken raw where possible, grated or juiced, and consumed in small quantities. Betacyanin in beetroot may cause red urine and faeces in some people who are unable to break it down. This is called 'beeturia', and the client should be warned of this possibility – it can otherwise be quite a shock when looking into the toilet bowl!

CRANBERRIES

Cranberries are a source of polyphenol antioxidants – types of phytochemical that are undergoing active research for their possible benefits to the cardiovascular and immune systems and as anti-cancer agents. Cranberry juice components have been shown to help prevent the formation of kidney stones. The tannins in cranberries have anti-clotting properties and may reduce urinary tract infections.

Cranberries and cranberry juice are abundant food sources of compounds which are powerful against human cancer cells in vitro, but their effect when taken by humans is as yet unproven. Nonetheless, since 2002 there has been an increasing focus on the potential role of cranberries in preventing several types of cancer. The berries also contain a chemical component that is able to inhibit and even reverse the formation of plaque by pathogens that cause tooth decay; they can even be used as a preventative for bad breath, because of their ability to fight oral bacteria!

There are several ways of taking cranberry, including juice, but several brands contain either sugar or aspartame as a sweetener and these should be avoided. Cranberry concentrate in tablet form is readily available and easy to take.

CHAPTER 15

Knee

The knee can be considered to be similar to the hamstrings in terms of the effects we are going to achieve. The knee itself is a joint made up of, and dependent on, the relationships around it. The muscles of the hamstrings reach down over the joint to grasp the tibia and fibula, and in like manner the muscles of the calf reach up to grab hold of the femur, in the catching-style wrist grip of a pair of trapeze artistes.

From a connective tissue perspective, the knee can be seen as being heavily influenced, from the outside and inside, by pressures and tensions placed on it by these various muscle and fascial connections. For example, a slightly inverted ankle will create a little more tensional strain along the lateral side of the leg, and therefore place more tension and potential strain on the knee as a result. Similarly, if we look at the lower back and gluteal area, then tension, shortening or postural deviations in the lower back and pelvis will create more tension in the knee. We can again draw an analogy between this and a hammock, and see that the joint sits in the centre between the ropes at either end.

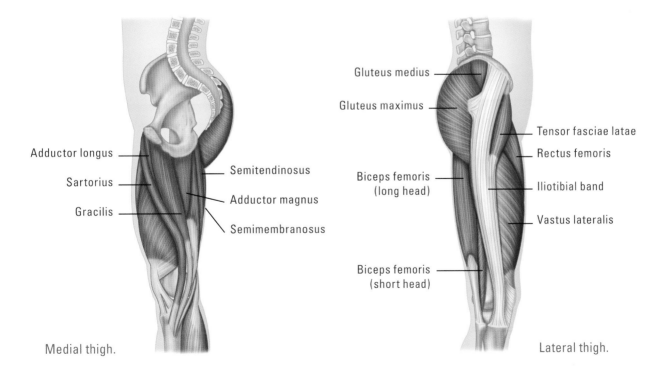

Medial thigh.

Lateral thigh.

In the traditional assessment of knee presentations, the knee is often addressed in isolation, which might not seem unreasonable. A knee which has damage to the meniscus, cartilage or ligament needs to be addressed and repaired, possibly surgically. However, from an integral bodywork perspective, the relationships to and from the knee are as important as the knee itself. We need to find out why it is that the problem has arisen and why the injury has occurred.

A common presentation will be a client who has experienced back trouble for years, and who has modified their weight bearing and movement patterns in order to adjust to the pain levels they experience. It is this compensation that causes conflict: uneven pressure, inequality of stance, uneven rotation or differences in movement all lead to unbalanced wear and tension in the lower limb. We've all seen someone standing with one leg forward, the pelvis pushed up and the weight being shifted across, and the other knee in hyperextension. It is a common sight and one which, over a period of time, will begin to set into the pattern of the body. Collagen fibres will continue to be laid down to support this function, and if injury were to occur once this pattern has been established, any attempt to isolate the problem to the specific injury will probably fail in the long term.

An argument often put to me is that it is impossible to avoid contact injuries in sports such as rugby and football. Of course, a violent tackle is highly likely to result in an injury to a specific area. Yet the level of injury, and therefore the speed of recovery, are going to depend a lot on the level of tension that was present at the site prior to the injury. A joint which is highly stressed as a result of a previous injury, or from tensions in other areas of the body above or below the site, will mean that any injury to the area will be potentially more serious. If the tensions in these areas are left unaddressed and only the injury site treated, then full recovery is unlikely. This in simple form is the case for preventative treatment of the whole body, and for full history taking to establish prior injuries. Moreover, a good therapist will be skilled in reading how a client holds their body and the patterns they use to move around.

CONTRIBUTING FACTORS

A knee might eventually even need replacing. However, it seems completely illogical to ignore the possible causative contributing factors at the same time as the knee is surgically addressed. Knees wear out for various reasons, but the human knee is more than capable of lasting 120 years without wearing out. However good the surgery, if it is being performed in the middle of an existing problem, the problem isn't going to go away.

It is vital to start by comparing one knee to the other and make as many observations as possible. How does the client stand, sit, cross their legs and take their shoes off? Ideally you would make these observations without the client being aware of it: a self-conscious client makes for very unreliable body-reading!

The influence of the ITB cannot be underestimated as far as the knee is concerned: ITB syndrome has been well established as a cause of knee pain, both in orthopaedic medicine and in the field of sports injury. However, as dissective evidence shows, the ITB is part of a wider structure of fascial covering around the leg, and palpation to determine other areas of tension can be useful in pinning down any other regions where the knee is being affected. Areas to palpate include the anterior compartment of the leg, where in many cases the fibres of the ITB extend down and seem to create a string-tension relationship between the foot and the thigh.

The patella can be seen as floating in a sea of connective tissue; it is embedded in a soft pad all the way around the knee and held in place by a ligament which also blends into the rest of the knee fascia. The knee influences a lot of other movement patterns throughout the body, acting as a mechanism for diverting forces through the back and into the upper body from the ankle, as well as acting as a feed-forward point for functional movement. It can be thought of as a barometer for the tensional environment of the lower leg, and worked as part of addressing the ankles, hamstrings and lower back. Any swellings or inflammations can be addressed with traditional remedies.

The first move of the knee, commonly referred to as 'hit the lat' (HTL), works the lateral inferior border of the vastus lateralis tendon, also known as the tendon of the quadriceps femoris. The move can be thought of as a complete treatment, as this point for the knee is very similar to the junction point of the superior medial angle of the shoulder (moves 6 and 8 of Page Two). At this point for working the knee, the ITB joins together with the vastus lateralis, the patellar ligament and the tendon of the quadriceps to become one large, tense and highly energetic covering around the knee. When dissecting this area, it is very difficult to single out where one structure begins and another ends, making the HTL a move that encompasses the whole of the knee. Many practitioners will also attest to the noise that is heard in the stomach when making this move, although it is not entirely established as to why this happens.

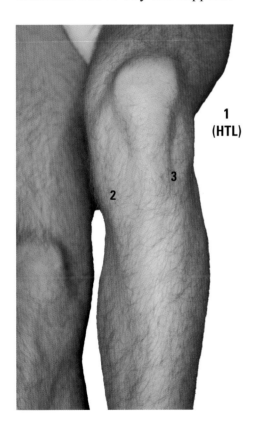
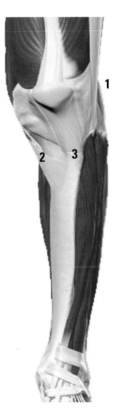

Location of the knee procedure moves 1–3.

Moves 2 and 3, which can be performed in any order, aim to lift the fatty pad that sits under and around the patellar, which in turn floats over the joint and takes pressure off the vastus intermedius, which is attached to the femur. The patellar ligaments are very deep under this structure, and once again the hammock analogy is dragged out to illustrate the moving aspect of the patella, held under tension by the ligaments at either end. The patella almost floats in the fatty tissue around the knee, which needs to have an appropriate degree of tension to keep the movements of the joint under control.

It is always worth moving the patella around to check its mobility. If it is stuck, the HTL will generally give it a degree of freedom quite quickly. If it remains stuck, and the 'lat' is sticky and hard to feel, gentle mobilisation of the patella will be helpful.

Moves 5 and 6, again in any order, roll around the lateral and medial heads of the gastrocnemius and soleus. These moves create a release for the posterior compartment of the leg, but also act strongly on the ankle joint where the gastrocnemius muscles join with the Achilles tendon and continue around the heel bone into the plantar fascia of the foot. The teasing moves along the back edge of the calf need to be done very gently for the best effect. These are not pulling or rolling moves, but a very gentle teasing action using the tips of the fingers.

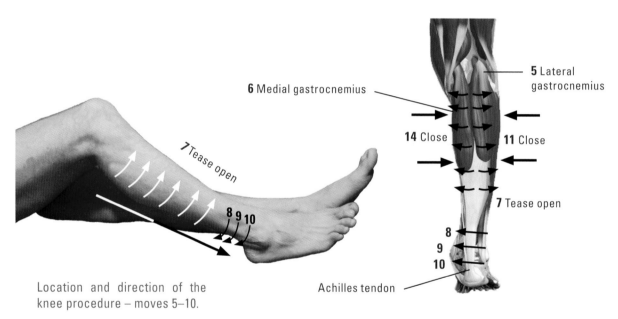

Location and direction of the knee procedure – moves 5–10.

In my experience a tender, swollen or inflamed calf responds to this gentle teasing much more quickly than any attempt to go in with depth and separate the muscles. Many exceedingly swollen legs have responded remarkably to these gentle teasing moves down the leg. Patience and plenty of breaks are the key to reducing any swelling; using force, or even much more than moderate pressure, is both counterproductive and potentially very harmful. We still have to bear in mind the sock-like aspect of the fascia underneath our fingers, which seems to be very responsive and sensitive to gentle touch. A swollen knee will also respond well to this teasing, and the three medial moves across the Achilles will help to release excess fluid into the medial side of the ankle to promote lymphatic movement.

The small move at the back of the malleolus can therefore be quite a useful addition to the knee procedure, especially if the ankle procedure is to follow or if there is any presentation of sciatic-type symptoms radiating into the ankle or foot. Although appearing somewhat complicated and fiddly, the knee procedure can be performed straight through with no break in cases where a preventative treatment is being given, and where there is no immediate or obvious problem.

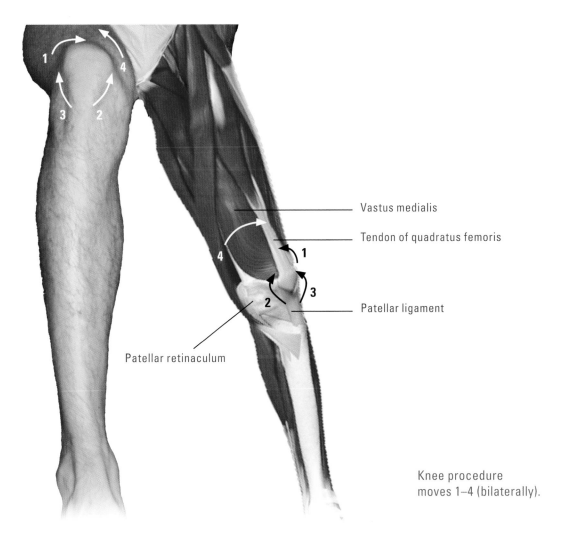

Vastus medialis

Tendon of quadratus femoris

Patellar ligament

Patellar retinaculum

Knee procedure
moves 1–4 (bilaterally).

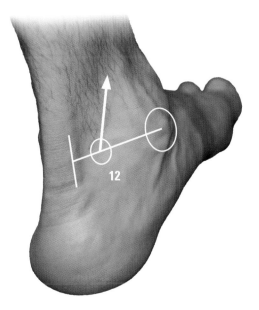

Location of the knee procedure
move 12 (tibial nerve).

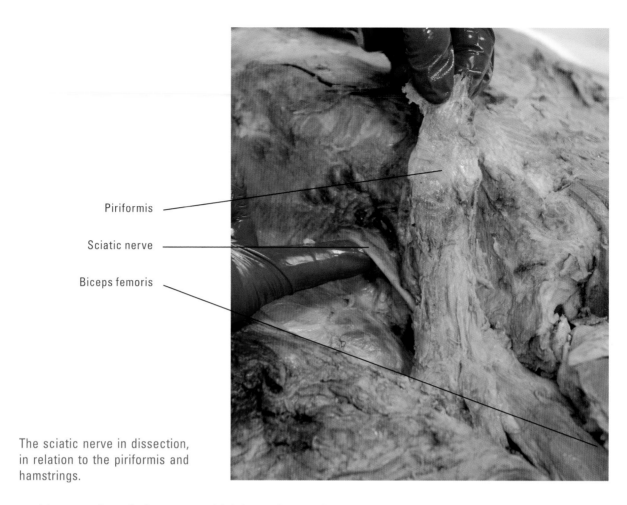

Piriformis

Sciatic nerve

Biceps femoris

The sciatic nerve in dissection, in relation to the piriformis and hamstrings.

A word here on the sciatic nerve, which is made up of two nerves – the tibial and common peroneal. As thick as your thumb and very sinewy, the nerve separates into its component parts around the back of the knee and travels down either side of the leg, sending off branches along the way. When the tibial nerve reaches the back of the medial malleolus, it divides into the medial and lateral plantar nerves. These nerves are responsible for quite a lot of innervation in the foot, and in turn can be indicated in a fair number of problems, including plantar fasciitis or pain in the sole of the foot.

CHAPTER 16

Pelvis

The pelvis procedure is generally considered the highlight of Bowen in terms of the effects that can be obtained with this relatively simple and quick treatment. In respect of relative effectiveness it is almost a complete therapy in itself, and there are many books in print about various pelvic presentations and treatments that could be shortened considerably by the use of this single procedure.

When we talk about the pelvis we need to define the area of reference for this. The three bones of the pelvic region are the sacrum, the hip bone (or innominate bone) and the femur. The coccyx could also be included in this section, fused as it is to the sacrum; this is not unreasonable and indeed brings in the pelvic floor grouping as another area which can be addressed with the pelvis procedure. The pelvis can be regarded as a major connective tissue junction which muscles and other connective tissues arrive at and depart from, with destinations as far away as the shoulder and ankle. Thus the pelvic area acts as a major stabiliser for the whole body.

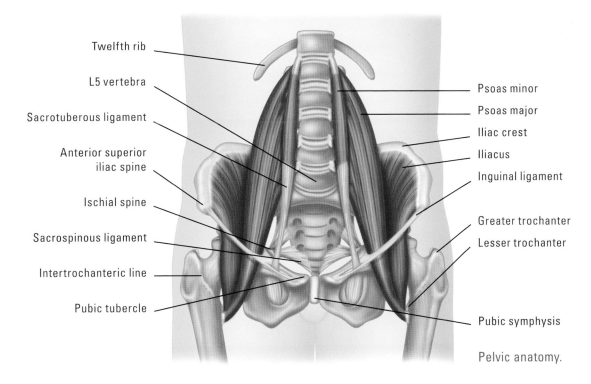

Twelfth rib

L5 vertebra

Sacrotuberous ligament

Anterior superior iliac spine

Ischial spine

Sacrospinous ligament

Intertrochanteric line

Pubic tubercle

Psoas minor

Psoas major

Iliac crest

Iliacus

Inguinal ligament

Greater trochanter

Lesser trochanter

Pubic symphysis

Pelvic anatomy.

There are many indications for using the pelvis procedure, some of which are not always obvious. A pelvic imbalance can often manifest in areas away from the problem, such as problems in the shoulder and neck, diaphragmatic and breathing conditions, and structural problems with the knee and ankle. Indeed, I will often claim that, given only three procedures to take to my desert island, I would choose the pelvis, knee and ankle, with of course the prerequisite Pages One, Two and Three.

The pelvis will present tilted (or 'out') to some degree in almost every client, and we need to decide, on an individual basis, whether this imbalance is a contributing factor in the problems the client is describing. There are four main imbalances that we can see in the pelvis:

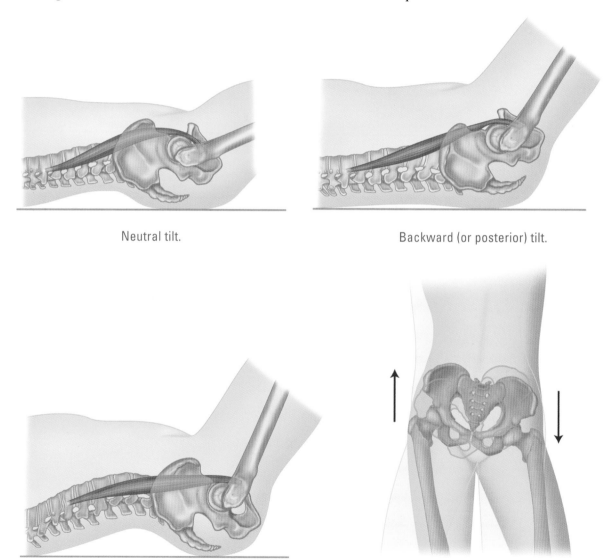

Neutral tilt.

Backward (or posterior) tilt.

Forward (or anterior) tilt.

Pelvic rotation.

The reasons for all of these, including the diagnoses and functions, constitute a subject which has filled many books, and isn't one we can fully address here, so a very potted version is called for. The most common presentation will be the lifted pelvis, which will create a leg-length difference. There are again many reasons for this, but commonly the condition is associated with an injury on one side to the hip, knee or ankle. Postural adjustment takes very little time, and someone spending three weeks limping or using a stick will adopt an uneven posture that may well have knock-on effects for injury or pain later on.

A leg-length difference will have mitigating factors all through the body, causing lower back, shoulder and neck pain, and even jaw problems. It is rare, however, for any kind of leg-length difference to really be a result of one leg being physically longer than the other. Instead, for a host of reasons, it is highly likely that one side of the pelvis is raised compared to the other. This could in turn be driven by a raised shoulder, which can frequently be seen after a shoulder injury.

Other factors might be involved in a pelvic tilt, particularly short or tight hamstrings, which might also be addressed at the same time, or considered if changes in the tilt are not occurring. The upper body is also involved with the position of the pelvis. If we refer to the connective tissue model, with the whole body being held in tension, then we can understand that elevating the shoulders, dropping the head or neck, or changing the position of the chest will each have a balancing requirement or change in the pelvis.

It is quite hard, however, to make the decision as to whether any elevation or tilt of the pelvis stems from the shoulders, the hamstrings or the pelvis itself – there are a lot of factors involved. An easy place to start, however, is to look at the client lying down, compared to them standing. Does the pelvis appear to be relatively level when they are prone and supine, but become lifted when they are standing? In this instance it is probable that the pelvic imbalance is coming from somewhere else. When someone is walking, if we can see that their shoulder moves or lifts before their legs or lower body, then this potentially indicates that the pelvis is being influenced by some imbalance in the shoulders.

I realise that this might all sound a little vague, with words such as 'potentially' and 'possibly' being used a lot. The trouble is that the human structure is remarkably adaptable and clever, and one which will compensate very quickly to achieve some degree of what can be considered normal. Think about it. You sprain your ankle and it really hurts. You don't sit in a wheelchair or lie in bed until the pain goes away, but instead you walk as best as you can, probably limping. It is this limp which is a very effective and powerful compensation. In a very short space of time, your body will start to adapt to that movement pattern, changing how you lift your pelvis, how you contract your buttocks and how you lift and move your shoulders and arms, not to mention your feet.

All these patterns that we have asked the body to take on are learned potential functional movements, available to us instantly, on file whenever we need them. In treatment situations we often see responses that entail the client experiencing pains that they haven't had for a long time. "The knee pain I had as a teenager came back overnight. I was in agony for about four hours." It is the body's way of exploring where you have stored information about all the compensations you have developed over the years. Call them coping mechanisms if you will.

It is not that these compensations are bad or wrong – quite the contrary. They demonstrate the immense range of strategies that the human body has at its disposal. The Internet abounds with stories of miracles, such as people paralysed from the waist down teaching themselves to walk and move again, seemingly normally; or feats of the mind controlling the body, as well as the body being able to take on, learn and rapidly adapt.

One of my favourite examples of this is the different heights of steps that can be found in old castles around the world. If you run up a flight of stairs, you don't think for a second how you manage to not trip up; an amazing and complex series of calculations is taking place in your body and brain, measuring, within two steps, the height of the next one. If you were going to develop a strategy to defend your castle, it would therefore make sense to make the steps irregular in height. Any invading soldier would run up the first two or three, then trip over the next one, slowing them down (as well as those behind) and giving you time to get the oil on the boil. The same approach can be found in the back stairs of country mansions, with purposely placed irregular steps to discourage the menial staff from running.

We can thus see the rapidity of adjustment that the body can take to alter the way it moves. This, I feel sure, is achieved via the changing tensions within the fascial tissues, with the brain and central nervous system following on behind. If this is the case, it also explains why and how we can see such rapid changes using a procedure like the one for the pelvis: four simple and quick moves can yield the most profound changes in what is a fairly complex structure. Yet, over and over again, we see long-standing leg-length differences, rotations, torsions and shifts changing almost immediately. This can of course happen with other hands-on therapies, but the difference is that, because with Bowen it is the client doing the work, the work holds and more work is often not needed.

CASE STUDY

It was December 21st and I had been asked to give a one-hour talk on Bowen to a group of graduating chiropractors. It was part of an awareness day of other therapies; I was sharing the day with a homeopath, a cranial therapist and a couple of others. I was last to speak. It was dark and a bit foggy, and everyone wanted to get away, so I decided to cut my talk short and spare everyone!

However, I did want to demonstrate the pelvis procedure. I spotted one lady who I could clearly see had a leg-length difference and postural issues as a result. On questioning she reported frequent back pain and aching. I asked the students to assess her pelvis for me, which took them quite a few minutes, finally putting forward an impressive array of issues that were present.

The pelvis procedure took no more than two minutes as a demonstration and treatment, preceded by the first four moves of Page One. I then asked the lady to get off the couch and walk around, before asking her to lie down again and instructing the assembled students to carry out a reassessment. They crowded around and muttered for quite some time, until someone raised their head and mournfully asked: "Why have I just spent four years studying chiropractic?" The lady's pelvic issues had been addressed almost immediately. These problems, which were long-standing and constant, stayed at bay until she returned to college in the New Year and was adjusted by a fellow student.

We also need to think of other areas into which the pelvis procedure can reach. The reproductive and urinary systems are heavily influenced by the pelvic treatment, on the basis that any imbalance in the pelvic area will create tension through the grouping of muscles that we refer to as the pelvic floor. For more information about the pelvic floor, refer to the coccyx section (p.73).

The diaphragm and transversus abdominis (TA) are strongly related via their attachments to the costal margin. Such is the strength of this relationship that Gil Hedley refers to the diaphragm and TA as 'transverse abdominalis verticalis', and the TA as 'transverse abdominalis horizontalis'. See the discussion of the diaphragm (Chapter 11) for more details. The diaphragm and TA overlay the next layer, the deep fascial bag containing the viscera. This is the parietal peritoneum and is held in tension all the way from the bottom of this bag to the top, as well as all the way around. This structure is explored in more detail in the diaphragm chapter, but the point here is that the bottom of the bag sits deep in the pelvis and has a strong relationship with its internal muscular structure, as well as a tensional relationship with the lower back and sacrum via the thoracolumbar fascia.

We can demonstrate this connection with a simple exercise. Take a breath and observe the quality and effort needed. Now squeeze the pelvic floor as if you are desperate to go to the toilet. At the same time as you squeeze, take another breath: is it harder or easier? If you have any degree of strength in your pelvic floor, the answer should be harder. This is simply because you are limiting the movability of the top of the diaphragm, making normal movement more difficult. From this we can see that even the breath has elements found in the pelvis, and purely from a 'standard anatomy' approach we know that the quadratus lumborum, which references to the posterior edge of the ilium, is a stabiliser for the diaphragm.

LYMPHATICS

The pelvis procedure is one of the indicated moves for addressing the lymphatic system, given the concentration of lymph nodes in this area. See the section on lymphatics for further information.

> **CAUTION**
>
> Clients with hip replacements must not have their hip extended past 90 degrees at any time.
>
> A condition of performing this procedure is that the client covers the genital area with his/her hand, and this must be preceded by an explanation. Use the ECBS photo guide as a demonstration tool if necessary.

APPLICATION

The prerequisite moves for the pelvis will generally be Page One; however, as a minimum, moves 1–4 of Page One would always be performed, with the HTL being performed to complete Page One when the client turns over.

The first move of the pelvis procedure is once again the HTL. Since this has already been done earlier, it might seem unnecessary now. However, the aim of the initial HTL was to link up all the moves performed for Page One, whereas for the first move of the pelvis procedure, the HTL is kept on the same side by the next three moves. This effectively means that, although the move is the same, the outcome and intention are different.

The second move is over the adductor longus (AL), and this warrants a cautionary word. The attachment of the AL is on the underside of the pubic bone, and for greatest effect the move should be performed as close to this location as possible. This means that if we are performing the move on a male, his genitalia will be sitting on the backs of our hands unless we ask him to move and hold them out of the way. With a female, we will also have our hands quite a long way up the thigh, and the placing of her hand over the genital area will protect both client and therapist.

There has been much discussion over the years about the wording to use with the client for this situation, but the advice is to be as matter of fact as possible about it and use whatever wording works for you. A therapist working in a rugby club might use a very different approach to a therapist in a general practice. What is most important, however, is that you try to be as confidentand comfortable as possible, as nerves and doubt on your part will quite likely create problems. It is suggested that you use the ECBS photo guide to show to your client, to inform them clearly what you are asking them to do. For more information, contact the European College of Bowen Studies at www.thebowentechnique.com

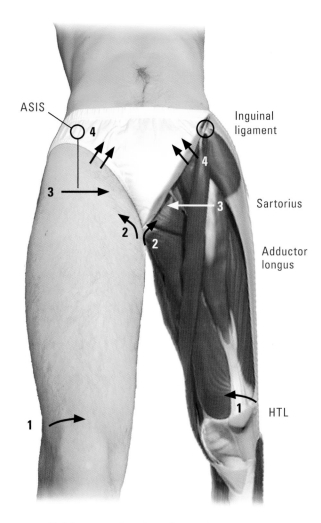

Pelvic procedure location and moves.

Because this area is generally well covered in tissue, it is important that we palpate to clearly identify the muscle, lifting the leg or contracting the adductor to feel this muscle under our fingers. When we have found it, we will also need to push the skin slack away and curve the fingers in order to get a good purchase on the posterior surface of the muscle. As with all Bowen moves, a curve is followed by a flattening of the fingers which should roll the muscle, and this action is one that needs practice to make perfect. I must emphasise that this move should not be painful! Whilst there will often be a degree of sensitivity in this area, the level of pain inflicted by some therapists that I have witnessed is not only pointless, but ultimately detrimental.

I am often asked whether this move is over the gracilis or the adductor longus. It is this kind of question that forces us to examine carefully what we do, where we do it and why we do it. The starting point in terms of answering the question is that it depends how far up the inside of the thigh you intend to do the work. The reason why we insist that the client places their hand over their genital area is that we want to work as close to the pubic bone as possible. If we are almost adjacent to the pubic bone, the division isn't so relevant, as the two muscles join together to become one, fairly well down from the supposed attachment. The anatomical pictures even suggest this, although the actual relationship is much clearer when revealed by dissection.

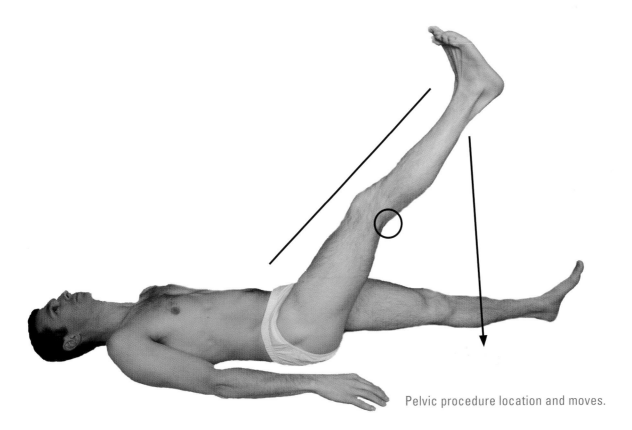

Pelvic procedure location and moves.

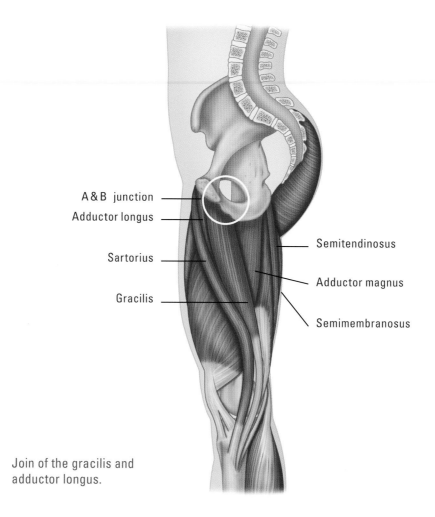

A&B junction

Adductor longus

Sartorius

Gracilis

Semitendinosus

Adductor magnus

Semimembranosus

Join of the gracilis and
adductor longus.

From a functional viewpoint the adductor, as its name suggests, is involved in adduction of the thigh, and makes up the anterior border of the pelvic triangle. In contrast, the gracilis is a fairly weak adductor and is primarily involved in flexion of the knee, in conjunction with the sartorius. As the sartorius is taken care of with move 3 of the pelvis, it stands to reason that the adductor longus is the main player in the pelvic move. If you get far enough up, however, it makes no difference anyway.

The higher up you carry out this move, the more effective you are likely to be. Bowen tends to isolate and aim for junctions where tissues conjoin, and where strong energetic and stress loading will create release. Work halfway along a muscle or a structure and you are as likely to hurt someone as you are to address the problem. A skilful therapist should feel the challenge of the adductor muscle and then be able to control its movement as it rolls backwards. Note the importance of short fingernails for the therapist!

While we are here, the psoas muscle deserves a few words. An awful lot has been written about the psoas major, much of it speculative and incorrect. Even more is suggested in relation to its treatment and palpation, and any attempt to touch the psoas must be done with extreme caution. The potential for causing damage and pain is, in my view, greater than any hypothetical outcome. Quite apart from anything else, in the Bowen world the procedure for the pelvis does as much as any other for balancing the psoas, without the need to go in deeply.

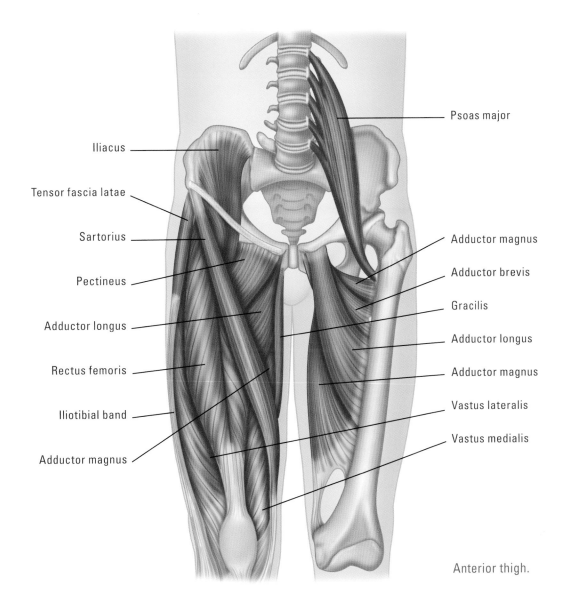

Iliacus

Tensor fascia latae

Sartorius

Pectineus

Adductor longus

Rectus femoris

Iliotibial band

Adductor magnus

Psoas major

Adductor magnus

Adductor brevis

Gracilis

Adductor longus

Adductor magnus

Vastus lateralis

Vastus medialis

Anterior thigh.

It is very difficult to palpate, with any degree of accuracy and clarity, the psoas muscle through the many layers of tissue covering it. During the dissection process, physical therapists with many years' experience have been surprised, and indeed dismayed, when shown the location of the psoas major muscle, sitting deep in the abdominal cavity or tucked back into the pelvis, and joining with the iliacus. The psoas major is more properly regarded as being primarily a stabiliser rather than, as more commonly thought, a flexor of the hip.

The third move is medially across the sartorius, the longest muscle of the body and the muscle which helps, via the flexion of the knee, in the action of crossing our legs, hence the label 'tailor's muscle' (sartor is Latin for 'tailor'). Also found in this area is the tensor fasciae latae (TFL) on the lateral edge and the conjoined tendon of the psoas major and iliacus. I am more and more convinced that the sartorius is a sling structure. The end point of the sartorius is always given as the anterior superior iliac spine (ASIS), yet its fascia is easy to follow around the edge of the ilium, continuing around into the lower back. It also brings into question what we mean when we talk about the inguinal ligament.

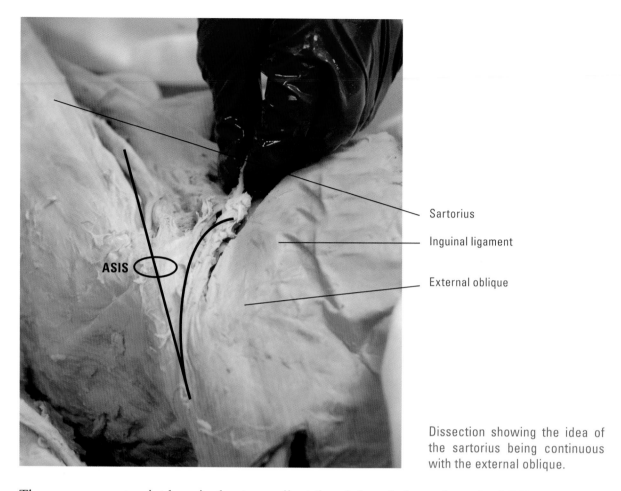

Sartorius

Inguinal ligament

External oblique

ASIS

Dissection showing the idea of the sartorius being continuous with the external oblique.

The measurement point here is about one client thumb-length down from the ASIS. Do not venture too low, as the sartorius runs diagonally towards the tibia: if you go too far down the leg, you'll miss it. Again, there needs to be some skin slack in this area. As with the adductor move, we need to be conscious of where our fingers are in relation to the genitals, and make any necessary adjustments, bringing the fingers into a fist if we find ourselves being invasive in this area.

The last move is across the inguinal ligament, which is effectively a combination of the fascia of the abdominal wall and the fascia of the thigh and ITB. The inguinal ligament stretches across from the ASIS to the pubic bone, and the femoral artery, nerve and vein run underneath it. The key here is that this ligament is not really a ligament at all, but a major tensional player in the stability of the pelvis and the pubic bone. The ligament proceeds over the pubic symphysis and into the corresponding ligament on the other side. In some instances this 'ligament' continues on to the surface of the ilium, creating a hoop effect over the pelvis and around into the lower back.

The fact that the tissues continue into the abdominal area means that an overworked, over-tense or overly 'stable' abdominal section could increase the tensional pull on the groin area where the inguinal ligament is located. Groin strains are common injuries in football players; however, also common in young, fit football players are highly developed rectus abdominis muscles, or cosmetically impressive, albeit pointless, six-packs. This will also have the unintended effect of increasing tension in the groin. Thus, when the leg or hip is externally rotated, say to pass a ball, and a tackle is taken, the potential for a groin injury is greatly increased.

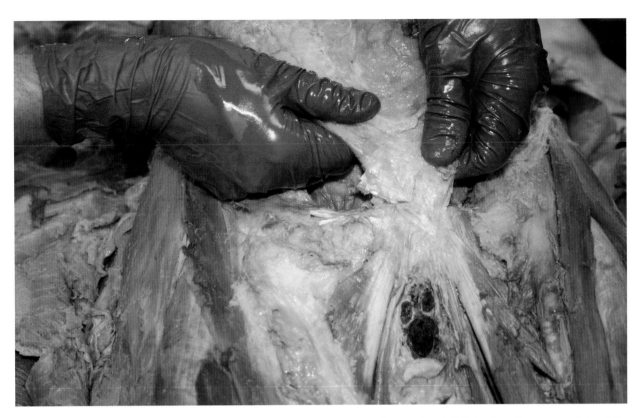

Dissection showing the continuous and strong nature of the adductor longus fascia joining into the rectus abdominis.

The index finger and middle fingers make this move; they should be slightly spread not only to avoid putting pressure on the femoral artery, but also to get a good spread along the ligament. As with the other two moves, it is important to have the fingers out of the way as the ring and little finger could easily find themselves being invasive. Lifting the leg during this move causes two things to happen: firstly, the extended tension on the ligament is relaxed, allowing palpation and movement of the tensioned tissue; secondly, gentle tension is created when the leg is pushed. The leg should be pushed towards the opposite shoulder when making this move, as this creates a pull through the sacrum and the sacrotuberous ligament, thus affecting the highly tensile structure of the sacrum and the sacroiliac joint.

When the leg is straightened, it needs to be extended as straight as possible, and as quickly as possible, without putting any stretch on the hamstring group, before being lowered to the table. All the structures of the sacrum and pelvis (including the psoas major and iliopsoas) are then addressed through the moves and the movement of the hip through the pelvis. A clicking sound, common in this area when lowering the leg, can be attributed to a number of things, one of which may well be the movement of ligament-type fascia over the edge of the ilium, around the sacroiliac (SI) joint and through the hip.

With little to compare their own skills to, it is often difficult for Bowen therapists to fully grasp the nature of what they are doing. The pelvis procedure is quite the crowning glory as far as Bowen is concerned and requires a lot of study and practice to get it perfect. It stands up in the field of bodywork as being a big player for presentations that are notoriously difficult, achieving consistently successful outcomes for very little investment. Learn it and look after it!

An alternative approach is to work the coccyx prone, with the pelvic moves added on the front, which produces interesting energetic changes to the pelvic floor and reproductive system; however, this will be explored in a future book. As with all Bowen 'procedures', there are variations on a theme and many ways that different presentations can be addressed. The intuitive therapist should therefore resist the model that proposes a 'this way is best' ideology.

SACRUM

Barely a day goes by without someone around us experiencing some level of back pain; this can of course vary from a slight niggle to a completely locked-up back. However, it is not always possible or practical to lay someone down and give them a treatment, but our desire to help them, as well as demonstrate the efficacy of Bowen, is nonetheless still there.

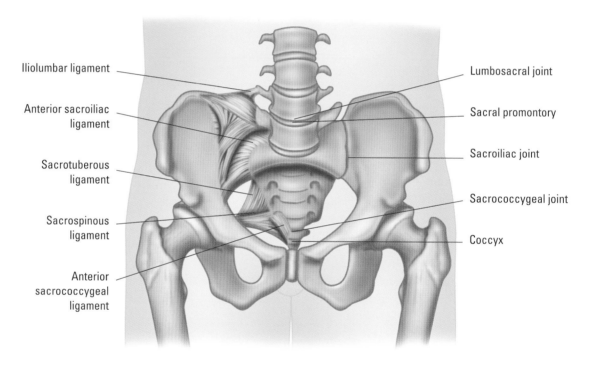

Iliolumbar ligament

Anterior sacroiliac ligament

Sacrotuberous ligament

Sacrospinous ligament

Anterior sacrococcygeal ligament

Lumbosacral joint

Sacral promontory

Sacroiliac joint

Sacrococcygeal joint

Coccyx

The ligamental structures of the sacrum.

The sacrum represents what I am coming to see as one of the most important areas of physical communication in the body. The suggestion is now that fascia acts as a feed-forward mechanism (Langevin, 2006) and a communicating network (Schleip, 2012). It therefore makes sense to look for a point in the body through which most structural tension is mediated and communicated. It is the sacrum that I would like to nominate for this location.

When looking at dissection in integral terms, that is, when looking for the connections rather than the separations, we can track a vast number of major (and minor) muscular structures to the sacrum.

As a joint goes, the sacrum itself isn't much of a mover: out of a possible 360 degrees of movement, it only manages about 4 degrees in any direction. However, it is lubricated just like any other joint, and held in place, particularly at the back, by an impressive network of connective tissues.

When considering the hamstrings (see Chapter 13), we saw how the sacrotuberous ligament connected up the head of the hamstrings to the sacrum. When attempting to find the attachment of the sacrotuberous ligament, however, the complexities of the sacral fascia make the distinction between the sacrotuberous ligament and the fascia of other structures virtually impossible.

From the end of the coccyx, the deep fascial connections of the muscles of the pelvic floor blend seamlessly into the anterior portion of the coccyx and into the deep fascia of the sacrum. To say that these simply 'attach' is just missing the nature of the whole relationship. In these same structures we see the attached fascial fibres of the piriformis, the gluteus maximus and minimus, and so forth. It is hard to really think of any muscle of the lower limb, trunk, lower back, mid-back, thorax, neck and shoulders that doesn't have a reasonably direct link to the sacral fascia.

The term 'thoracolumbar fascia' (TLF) is supposed to include the sacral fascia, shown as a sheet of fibrous material that covers the deep muscles of the back of the trunk. Even with the three well-established layers of this material, however, there is still a world of coverings and attachments that are not strictly encompassed by the term TLF.

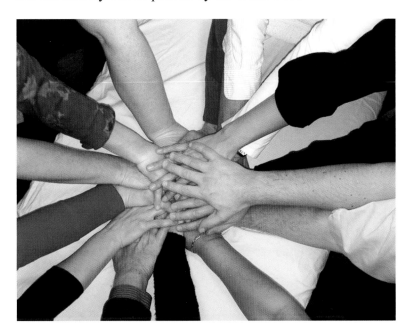

This complex and highly tensile region can be explained by visualising lots of hands piled on top of each other as shown in this picture. It does not really matter which way is up and which way is down here. The principle is that if a hand pulls at the bottom, then all the other hands will feel this pull. If another hand anywhere in the pile starts to move in any direction, this movement will be felt by all the hands, including the original deeper pulling hand.

It is this complexity of movement and information transmission through the sacrum that leads me to think of it as a movement and information mediator. Held in a massive amount of multidirectional tension, the sacrum creates a central balance and focus for movements from the lower to the upper body, and vice versa. In attempting to stand up from a sitting position, we bend forwards at the waist, lining up all the key levers through the ankles, knees, sacrum, neck and head. If, just before we stand up, we move our head back, even slightly, then standing up becomes impossible. By concentrating, we can feel that it is indeed the sacrum that is acting as a master of ceremonies for all this to take place.

The reasons for the sacral area going into spasm are many fold, and the procedure itself takes into account much of the traffic that goes through the area. Accuracy here is probably less important than in many other procedures, and the sacrum procedure can be performed more than once, with appropriate breaks, in the same session.

A word here about guiding the client to a standing position. It seems logical to suggest that the client might wish to stand as evenly as possible once the sacrum moves have been performed. Make sure, therefore, that you help the client up afterwards. Have them bend their knees, and place one hand on their collarbone and the other on their sacrum at the back. They can then stand, straightening their legs and using their knees to push up. This both minimises the level of pain they might experience and prevents them from twisting away from the side of the pain, thus avoiding the imbalance they arrived with. After the procedure, movement is very important: make sure the client moves around the room as much as possible, especially before trying the procedure again.

Some years ago I was invited to spend a few days treating staff and inmates of the prison ship HMP *The Weare* in Portland Harbour, Dorset. A large prisoner who had injured his back in the gym was about to be transferred to the local hospital, because of his level of pain and the fact that he was a fire risk, being unable to move freely around the narrow ship. I was given half an hour, during which I learned several new words from him and some information about my mother to which I had not previously been privy! However, it was when I got this man up and worked on him while standing, encouraging him to move around between sets of moves, that he started to respond. By the end of the session, his pain had subsided to the point that he was able to move freely, although he was issued with a walking stick. When I saw him a few days later he was exceedingly grateful, and apologetic for some of the more choice phrases he had chosen in order to express himself; but most importantly, he was free of pain.

The procedure is in essence very simple to perform, and even severely locked-up backs have responded instantly to the four simple moves involved. There are no contraindications for this procedure, but it is a good idea to make sure that the surface onto which the client is going to bend is one that they will be able to get back up from. When performing these procedures, you should try to work the better side first, if you can identify one, and, wherever possible, convince the person to come for a proper treatment as soon as possible.

There are hundreds of stories of Bowen therapists using this procedure in the most unusual and unlikely situations – from aeroplanes, bars and bus queues to doctors' waiting rooms. The response is generally one of disbelief, followed by amazement. Make sure that you stand to the side, where the client can clearly see you, and that your hands are not in a position in which they would be invasive or hang down onto the client's buttocks. In addition, although our model is wearing little in the way of covering, there is no real need to loosen any clothing or to lower trousers; however, with a client in tight jeans, the move can be challenging, to say the least, but still effective.

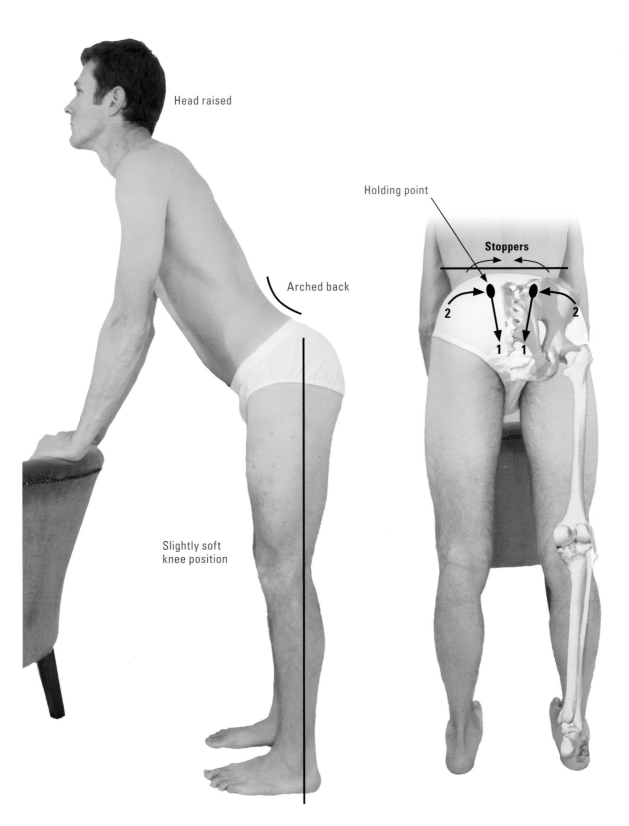

Head raised

Arched back

Slightly soft
knee position

Holding point

Stoppers

2

2

1   1

Position for performing the sacrum procedure – lateral view.

Sacrum position.

CHAPTER 17

Shoulder

The shoulder joint is the most mobile joint in the human body. This is mainly because, now that we are the only mammal to stand upright, we no longer need our upper limbs to be weight bearing. However, at the same time as the joint being incredibly mobile, it is also potentially fragile and can be injured and dislocated relatively easily, especially during certain sporting activities.

Anatomically, the major player in terms of the movement of the shoulder is of course the deltoid, but we need to look at this muscle in relation to other attachments and bony structures if we are going to be successful in working with problem shoulders. The traditional anatomical explanation of the deltoid indicates it attaching to the inferior angle of the spine of the scapula, with the trapezius attaching to the upper side of the spine. This does not really give a complete picture, however: from a fascial perspective, the attachments of the deltoid and the trapezius are more direct.

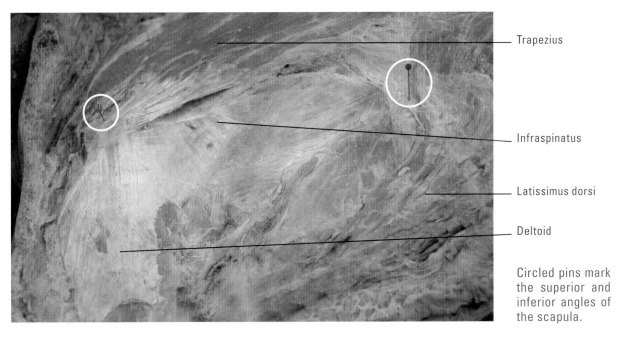

Trapezius

Infraspinatus

Latissimus dorsi

Deltoid

Circled pins mark the superior and inferior angles of the scapula.

The three aspects of the deltoid muscle – anterior, middle and posterior – take care of the various gross functions of the arm, namely flexion and extension, with the muscles of the rotator cuff being involved in rotation.

As well as attaching to the spine of the scapula at the back, the deltoid also has substantial attachments to the scapula at the front, on the acromion, and even on the medial edge, as the muscle blends in fascially with the infraspinatus. However, as we have already seen, the fascia of the deltoid also has a fairly strong relationship with the trapezius and the levator scapulae: these all form a strong bond at the superior medial angle of the scapula. Hence the importance of the 'lady bird' moves around the superior medial angle of the scapula.

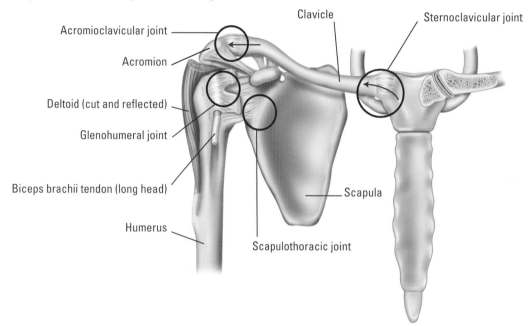

The implications for this are far reaching, but the first port of call is to understand that both shoulders are a complete unit and must be addressed as such. Because of the integral nature of the trapezius sitting across the whole of the upper back, any movement on one side, particularly an internal rotation of the shoulder, will have a follow-on effect on the other side. Because much of this movement will be mediated through the scapula, the moves of Page Two on the edge of the scapula are almost essential as a prerequisite for any moves performed on the rest of the shoulder.

In the lower part of the body, the latissimus dorsi attaches to the thoracolumbar fascia and the edge of the ilium, and acts as a powerful extensor of the arm. Therefore, if we are seeing the lower-back fascia shortened, the pelvis rotated or tilted, and/or the shoulders pulled accordingly, there is clearly the need to address the lower back before proceeding with the rest of the shoulder work: a case for referring to the initial moves if ever there was one.

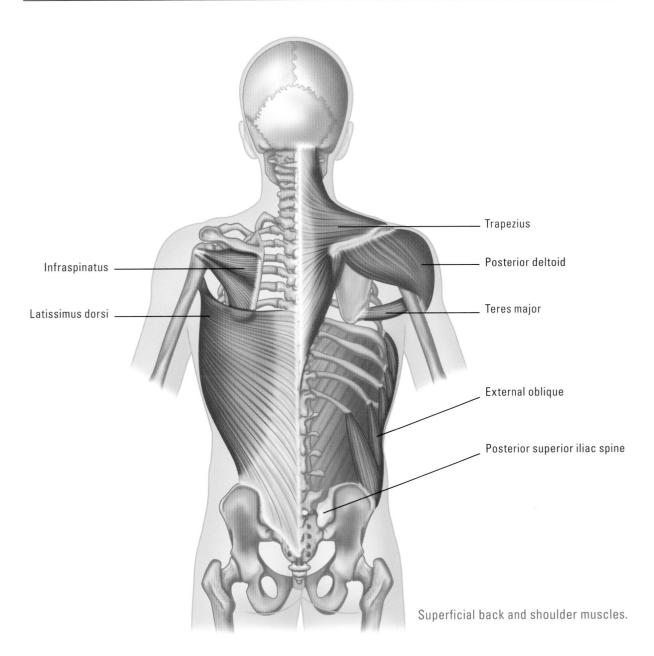

Infraspinatus

Latissimus dorsi

Trapezius

Posterior deltoid

Teres major

External oblique

Posterior superior iliac spine

Superficial back and shoulder muscles.

At the front of the body, the traditional view of the pectoralis major being separate from the deltoid is a puzzling one. In a dissection, the division between these two muscles is hazy at best and could be more accurately referred to as the 'deltopectoral groove' or 'pectoid'. The only way a separation can be achieved in order to create the image traditionally referred to is by cutting.

Therefore, from a tensional perspective, what we have is the deltoid and the shoulder joint being held in movement between the pectoralis at the front and the muscles adjoining the scapula at the back. To make matters even more complicated (or more interesting, depending on your perspective), the latissimus dorsi muscle connects the inside of the shoulder to the lower back. This gives stability to our shoulder movements, but also suggests that, with any shoulder restriction, the lower back or sacrum will need to be considered. I say 'considered' here rather than specifically stating that it should be treated, as each client is going to present differently; it is just something to consider.

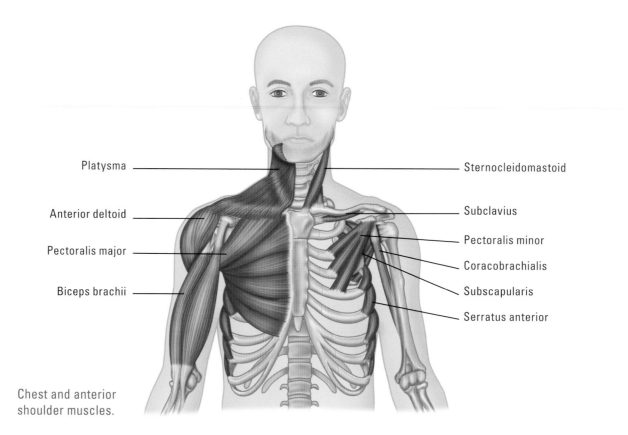

Platysma

Anterior deltoid

Pectoralis major

Biceps brachii

Sternocleidomastoid

Subclavius

Pectoralis minor

Coracobrachialis

Subscapularis

Serratus anterior

Chest and anterior shoulder muscles.

The attachments of the deltoid and the clavicle to the acromion, and the attachment of the pectoralis major to the clavicle, create a synergistic junction around the whole of the shoulder. This means that there are a lot of potential areas that could be considered or involved when addressing shoulder problems.

In terms of standard bodywork, the shoulder procedure is quite revolutionary, given the speed of efficacy and the simplicity of the move. Traditionally, with shoulder complaints it can be very difficult to get a response to conventional treatments, and surgery is frequently an option in difficult cases. A standard 'frozen shoulder' is now more commonly referred to as 'painful shoulder syndrome' and can encapsulate dozens of different presentations. 'Adhesive capsulitis' is another common name given to this condition, although it can often be referred to as such without any evidence of either adhesions or inflammation of the joint capsule. However, none of this causes much concern to the Bowen therapist. A client presenting with pain in the shoulder, limitation of movement, however severe, and/or referred pain into the neck or arm is a prime candidate for the shoulder procedure.

The shoulder procedure can also be used to assist in addressing other issues, including respiratory dysfunction, elbow, arm and wrist problems (such as carpal tunnel syndrome), and neck restrictions. The move itself is very simple in its application, but not the easiest to perform: because the move is being made with one hand while the other is carrying the client's arm, it can be tricky for the therapist to co-ordinate both of these operations. Traditionally, this move is performed with the help of an assistant who holds and carries the arm while the therapist makes the moves. In an ideal world this would be how we would treat every shoulder, but few of us can afford the luxury of an assistant on call whenever we need one. Instead, the move has been adapted to enable the therapist to perform it solo; the technique is still just as effective, but requires a good deal of practice to perfect.

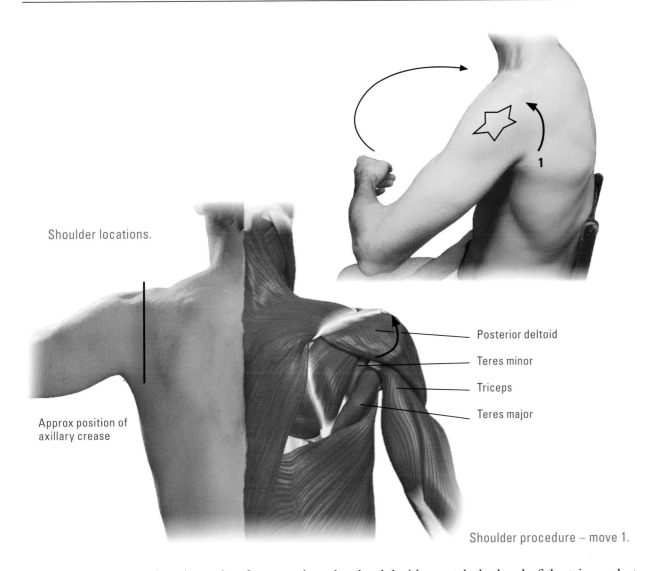

Shoulder locations.

Approx position of axillary crease

Posterior deltoid

Teres minor

Triceps

Teres major

Shoulder procedure – move 1.

The key to the procedure is getting far enough under the deltoid to catch the head of the triceps, but also taking in the fascial components of the teres major and minor and the subscapularis. The easiest way to find this point is to follow the line created by the axillary crease, which defines the separation between the shoulder and the arm. Timing and position are crucial to the success of the shoulder move, and the arm should be held by the therapist (or assistant) at an angle of slightly less than 45 degrees, with the elbow at around chest or breast height. Leverage to achieve the move is essential: while the move is being made with the middle and ring fingers, the thumb needs to be on the top of the shoulder, creating the leverage.

The move should be made while the arm is in motion, being carried towards the opposite shoulder, where the elbow needs to be pushed across to create a fairly firm tension through the shoulder girdle. If the client is sitting on a table, the pressure required to push the elbow across will be sufficient to push them off the table; if the move is going to be performed solo, it must therefore be made with the client sitting on a chair. The jar is made with the arm pushed all the way across and is into the stretched capsular tissue of the joint. This is an important element, as it somehow seems to return the shoulder joint to a 'default' setting. Indeed, even long-standing shoulder restrictions have been commonly restored to full range of motion after just one treatment using this procedure.

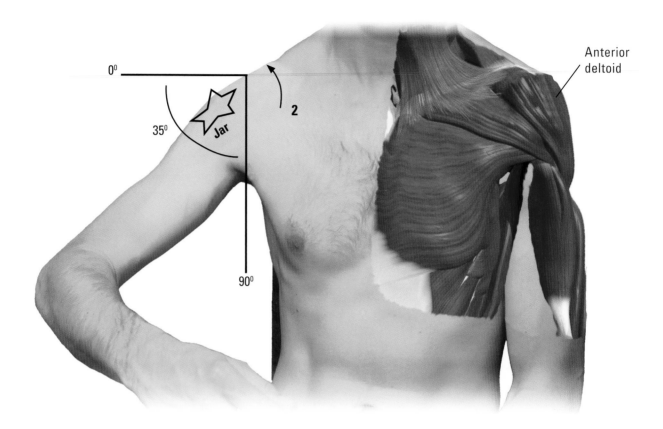

Shoulder procedure – move 2.

28-DAY RULE

The general rule of learning a physical movement is that it will take approximately three weeks of repetitive activity in order for the brain and body to start to accept a new pattern. This is true for negative as well as positive changes, so a three-week limp, for example will set up patterns of adjustment throughout the whole body. In order for the shoulder work to be absorbed and accepted as a new functional model, as well as avoiding inflammation of a very susceptible area, the shoulder procedure is only performed twice in two weeks, and time is then allowed for the changes to occur.

In the case of re-injury, the work can be repeated, and other areas of possible interest can also be treated in that time. For instance, the TMJ and the pelvis (Page Three) would both be areas that might need work if the shoulder is going to be fully addressed. Pages Two and Three would always be performed prior to a shoulder treatment wherever possible. The better side is treated in order to set up a touch response rather than a pain response. This is generally the rule of thumb throughout all Bowen treatments: treat the better side first where possible.

SHOULDER EXERCISES

The two standard exercises that have been taught for many years alongside the Bowen Technique shoulder moves are still as valid and relevant now as they ever were. This is not to say that there aren't many more exercises out there, but that these particular two are fairly simple to demonstrate and perform, quite easy to remember and very effective if performed regularly and correctly.

When giving any kind of aftercare advice, remember the principles of keeping it simple. I think of myself when it comes to being a client and how much I either listen or take in: however much I believe I will remember, I'm going to forget most of what I've been told before I get home!

The client doesn't need to know what you know, so keep things to a minimum and make it easy for the client to remember and actually do what it is you are asking them to do.

Demonstrate the exercises yourself, and then get them to do it with you. This will enable them to feel confident they are doing it right and know how it feels. Write things down for them wherever possible, making a note of what you've written. These notes act as reminders for both you and the client.

The information that comes back from a client is often unreliable. They are going to come back and tell you that they did the exercise every day, when in fact they only did it twice. They will also say that nothing has changed. Keep a good record of how they were presenting and the markers that go with this. In this way you will be able to rely on your own information, rather than on the sketchy details that clients will offer you.

Exercises, like stretches must never be done into pain. The idea is to gently mobilise the tissues and affected areas of the shoulder, not to create more pain or a problem. These exercises can also be performed as warm-up movements before participating in sports, particularly golf.

SHOULDER CIRCLES

The first exercise is a simple arm rotation through 360 degrees, range permitting. Starting with the arm hanging to the side, lift the arm forwards and upwards as far as possible. Try to allow the arm to pass through a complete arc at the top and then begin to reach behind, to allow the arm to come downwards through a full circle. If the arm cannot reach all the way to the top, allow it to go to a position before the point of pain, then come out of the circle.

Each circle is performed five or six times or until any before point of discomfort or aching arises. The circles must then be performed with the other arm.

Watch the client perform the circles and keep an eye on the shoulder to make sure it isn't lifted too soon. The shoulder blade and trapezius area shouldn't be lifting before the arm is at about chest or breast height, as this will limit the range that is possible. If the client has quite a severe restriction, this exercise can also be done leaning forwards and drawing circles on the floor, as if stirring a big imaginary pot of porridge.

SHOULDER ROTATIONS

The client can perform this movement when and if they are able to raise their arm to shoulder height without over-engaging the shoulder blade or trapezius. The exercise is designed to place gentle pressure on the shoulder capsule and increase movement and strength.

Stand side-on to a wall (or doorframe) and put one hand against the wall. You should be able to push against the wall, but should not be leaning into it.

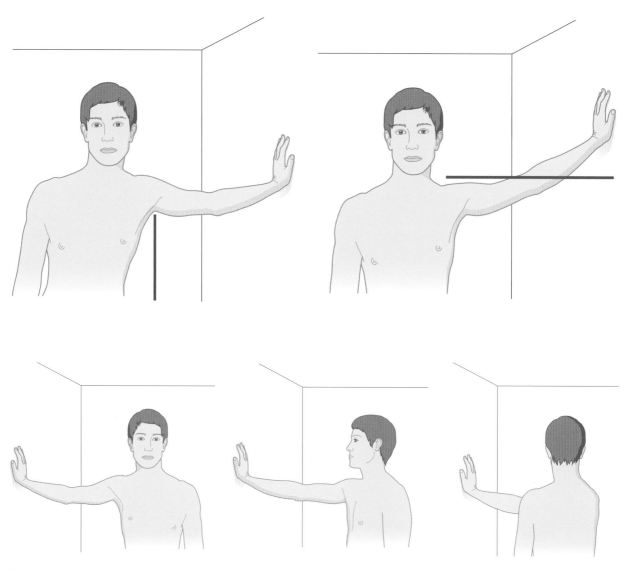

Correct starting position.

Keeping the arm still and straight, start to walk inwards towards the arm until it is against your chest. Again stop if there is any pain or discomfort in the joint or arm.

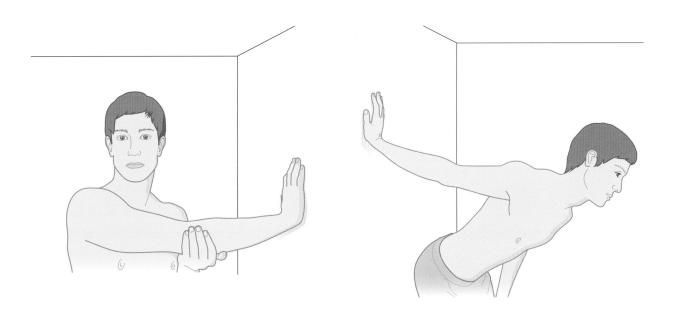

You can use the opposite hand or wrist to keep the elbow straight and hold the arm in place against the wall.

Hold this position for three seconds. Keeping your hand in contact with the wall, walk back in the direction you came from, but keep going. Eventually you will be facing the opposite direction to your hand and the wall.

Now bend at the waist and walk slowly backwards, until your bottom reaches the wall, with the arm above you.

NECK STRETCH

Shoulders are inextricably linked to the head and neck: a client with poor lateral flexion in the neck as well as restricted shoulder function will need to address the neck as a major part of getting the shoulders moving.

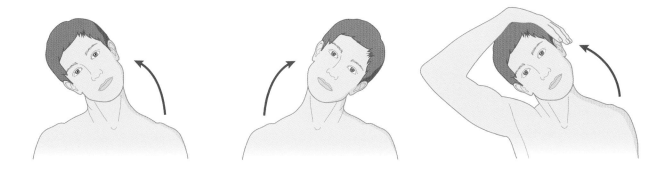

The neck can be stretched out very gently using just the weight of the head. The head should drop to the shoulders without being forced, and both sides should be stretched on a regular basis.

CHAPTER 18

Temporomandibular Joint

From a Bowen perspective, the temporomandibular joint (TMJ) procedure is one of the most important and powerful moves that we have. Yet it remains very misunderstood and also much underused, particularly when some of the presentations don't appear at first sight to be directly linked to the jaw. Nevertheless, the unique nature of the mandible and its association with the skull implicate it in hundreds of possible areas, from the top of the head to the tips of the toes.

The nature of the TMJ and the Bowen moves associated with it represent quite a complex structure surrounding what is effectively a very simple joint. It is difficult to know where to start when talking about the TMJ, such is the breadth of its inclusiveness. The TMJ is the most widely used joint in the body: every time you swallow, talk, chew and open your mouth you use this joint. Clicky jaws, facial pain and even some dental issues can often be addressed with the TMJ procedure, but other areas of the body will also be discussed in this chapter.

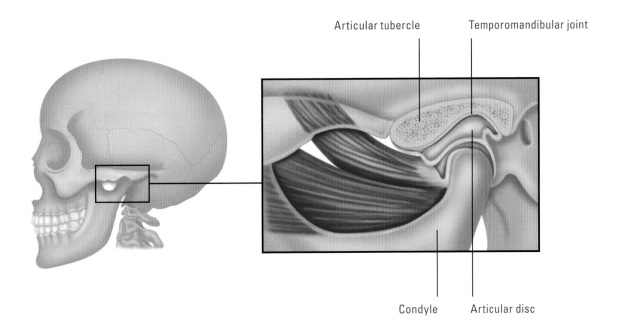

Articular tubercle   Temporomandibular joint

Condyle   Articular disc

There are two parts to the TMJ procedure, both of which are performed at the same time. The first element addresses the soft tissues of the face and the front of the neck; it starts the process of drainage by gentle milking of the lymph nodes behind the sternocleidomastoid (SCM) muscle. The second part is performed with the client gently biting the knuckle of their index finger, which creates a small stretch across the joint. The moves over the area adjust the position of the joint and release tension through the rest of the face and head.

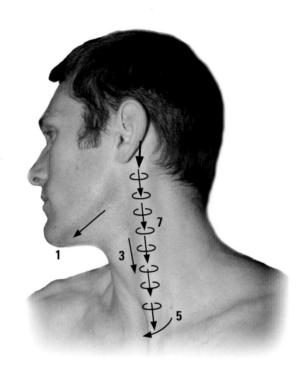

SCM drainage.

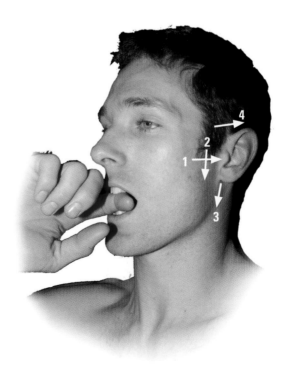

TMJ moves.

As well as addressing issues arising in the face and jaw, the TMJ also has implications for the rest of the body. The head weighs in the region of 6 to 7 kg, and the slightest movement away from centre will require the rest of the trunk to stabilise and counterbalance. The neck and shoulders are constantly working to accomplish this stability, and several important structures associated with the TMJ are in continuity with the neck and shoulders. The SCM muscles attach to the head onto the mastoid process of the skull, which is part of the temporal bone. Fascially, the SCM carries on around the scalp fascia and into the SCM on the opposite side, effectively creating a sling around the back of the head. Given that the SCM is a flexor of the neck and head, the implications for a resulting flexion in the rest of the trunk are fairly prevalent. The pushing of the weight of the head forwards with the flexion of the SCM, together with the flexing of the rectus abdominis, can easily create the potential for an overly flexed posture.

As humans have evolved, the act of standing upright has demonstrated their superiority over the animal kingdom. No longer do we need to lope around, ape-like, protecting our vulnerable areas – the groin, stomach and throat – from attack. Our evolution has taken us to the top of the food chain, and with our opposable thumbs and big brain, we no longer have any natural predators. Instead we can stand upright and survey the world around us. It is not, however, a very good position from which to either run away or defend ourselves, and this fully extended posture can only be achieved in the confidence that we are fairly safe.

Yet our natural safe position is in flexion. We spend nine months in the womb curled up in a flexed position, and many of us sleep naturally in the foetal position. We use expressions that reflect this to indicate safety and comfort, for example 'curled up on the sofa' and 'curled up in front of the fire'. This act of curling up represents cosiness, comfort and safety, and is an easy position to get into. Threat in a modern society is for the most part not a physical one. Whilst it is always possible, I feel it is unlikely that one would see someone curled up on the workplace floor after having been criticised or otherwise challenged by a workmate or employer … actors aside.

The same expressions of curling up, however, can also be used to express extreme emotional discomfort. "I could have curled up and died with embarrassment" is an example, suggesting that this curling reflex takes us to a point of safety, the starting point of this being from the head forwards. A position of servitude and humility, as well as depression and mental illness, the forward stoop into flexion is also a posture of deference. You might bow to royalty, or may have once upon a time tugged your forelock to the lord of the manor as a gesture of knowing your place. The potential for us to be able to breathe in this position was looked at in the discussion of the diaphragm in Chapter 11, but needless to say it is a difficult position from which to function.

The SCM also shares the TMJ site with the splenius capitis, the muscle that gives shape to moves 5 and 6 of Page Three and acts like a supporting bandage around the back of the neck. These superficial yet highly tensile structures are encased within a single layer of tight fascia which spreads over the head and blends across into the temporalis muscle. The SCM fascia, rather than 'attaching' to the mastoid process, is strongly blended and connected (referenced) with the fascia of the scalp – the galea aponeurotica – and works itself all the way over the head, blending into the strong fibrous tissues of the temporalis. The implications for the scalp fascia and the SCM being so strongly connected are far reaching. Symptoms such as headaches, migraines and upper body pain may well have origins in the lack of functional movement through the fascia of the scalp and therefore the SCM. The other muscle referencing through the mastoid is the posterior digastric, which facilitates depression of the lower mandible and is particularly active when chewing.

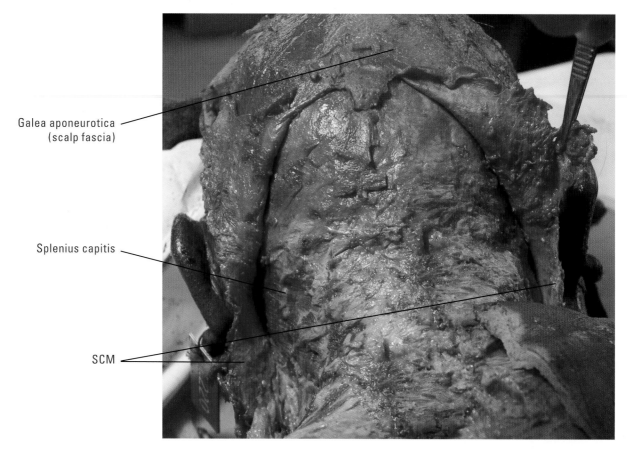

Galea aponeurotica
(scalp fascia)

Splenius capitis

SCM

This dissection shows the continuous nature of the SCM fascia with the scalp fascia. The SCM has been released from the mastoid bone, but at this point it is thick and its surface continues into the galea aponeurotica.

The relationship between the neck and shoulders and the TMJ work is important for several reasons. The first one, as already mentioned, is that much of the stability and counterbalancing for the head is going to come from this area. We can frequently observe imbalance by looking at the way a client lies supine on the couch: if their head is tilted to one side, or if their chin points away to their feet, then these are the positions that the body thinks are normal. On rising, adjustments will have to be made through the rest of the frame to create the sensation of being upright and straight.

This is the type of compensation to which I refer a lot when teaching and writing. Compensation causes conflict, and, in terms of pain and dysfunction, it is the conflict which will tend to present as the problem. If we don't address the compensation, however, which is likely to be well away from the site of pain, we will never have the opportunity to fully restore the original function – hence the frequency of footballers and athletes constantly re-injuring themselves.

The common posture of pushing the head and neck forwards, or over-flexion of the trunk, will mean that muscles and structures around the head will start to create a tensional draw which is unlikely to be even and will need to be balanced somewhere in the structure. This can often be seen in the lumpy, tissuey area at the top of the thoracic spine, sitting there as a counterbalance to an overly flexed or pushed-forward posture. The other area which might be used to compensate could be the lower back, with the strong fibres of the lumbar area creating a tensional balance, preventing us literally from falling flat on our faces.

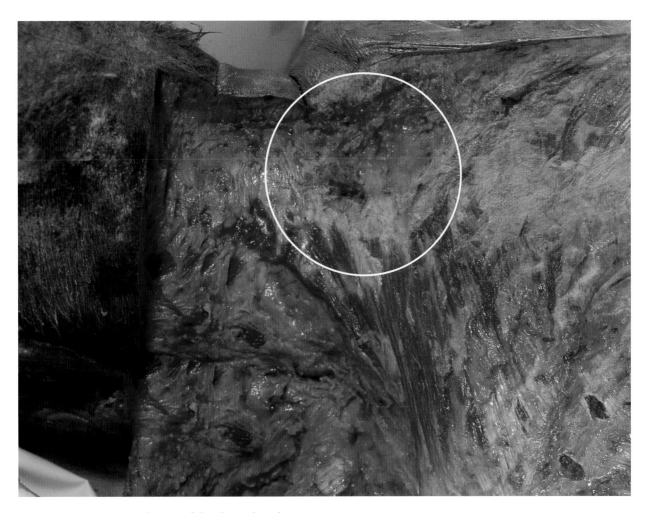

Lumpy, tissuey area at the top of the thoracic spine.

The TMJ needs to be referenced with the shoulders and arms as well, because of the big bundle of nerves serving the arm, neck and shoulders – namely, the brachial plexus – rising from the cervical spine and out across the top of the neck. The upper trunk comes out just behind the SCM and can be palpated without difficulty. A laterally flexed neck, as a result of a shortened or tight SCM, can easily place excessive pressure onto these nerves, creating carpal tunnel syndrome symptoms, arm and wrist pain, and presentations such as tenosynovitis.

The TMJ is also indicated with regard to respiratory dysfunction. The SCM attaches to both the sternum and the clavicle and is an important accessory muscle of respiration. A flexed, drawn-forward position will also create a limitation in terms of the ease of breathing and the function of the diaphragm. As discussed in the diaphragm chapter, posture is an essential part of functional breathing, and anything that will affect this needs to be addressed.

It is important to gauge the movement of the face and head before starting the TMJ procedure, not just to obtain functional markers but also to see whether other factors are involved with any imbalances. The first moves address the submandibular gland, which produces most of our saliva. It is a good place to start for people who are presenting with difficult swallowing, and links in with the hyoid muscles and with the whole of the digestive system.

Further along the neck, the separation between the trachea and the SCM is felt, with inferior moves over the inferior aspect of the SCM tendon being the last of this small set of moves. At its lower edge, the SCM continues into the fascia of the pectoralis, and at a deeper level into the chest wall, involving itself in respiration and linking all the way down to the pubic bone at its lowest point. The SCM has a significant involvement in the way that the lower back is held and in general posture and function.

The main advantage of using the head as a key point from which to start body reading is that it is always visible. Even if you put a sack over someone's head, you would still be able to see the position of the head in relation to the rest of the body, and establish whether the head is pushed overly forward. The drainage of the SCM shouldn't be viewed as simply drainage, but also as a relaxation of the actual muscle, which is working hard to keep the head on the shoulders. The skiing accident I mentioned earlier put all the SCM muscles into focus and was an excellent lesson on how every movement of the head and neck is referred around the SCM.

TMJ PROCEDURE

The breakdown of the TMJ procedure into two parts makes sense as long as it is understood that they can be applied separately as well. Someone presenting with reasons why you might not want to carry out the TMJ procedure could still happily receive the drainage elements quite safely. Before performing the TMJ procedure over the condylar heads of the joint, you should also check to make sure you are in the right spot, that is to say in the space between the zygomatic process and the head of the mandible.

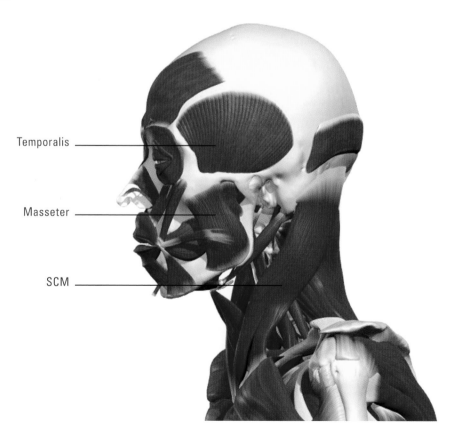

Temporalis

Masseter

SCM

The position of the fingers should be such that you can feel the movement of the joint and the ligament, without your fingers being moved by the action of opening and closing the jaw. The space here is tiny and the margin for error very small; once you are in the correct location, you should avoid taking the fingers away. It is at this point that the client is asked to put their knuckle between their teeth, biting gently down while the first two moves are performed over the joint. The order of the moves is of little importance here, but by moving posteriorly and inferiorly over this area, it will be ensured that the multiple tensions of this powerful joint are addressed. It is important to keep the fingers on both sides of the head in contact with the joint, as a small reading from one side to the other can often be felt as the moves are made.

The third moves are at the back of the mandible and are the closest moves to the vagus nerve that can be made. This area is also covered with the parotid gland and can be very sensitive, so care should be taken.

The final move in the sequence addresses the back edge of the temporal muscle and fascia. This tightly bound muscle sits under a thick fascial bag and also under the scalp fascia, which in turn is under pressure from the SCM. The temporal muscle also contains branches of the facial nerve at this point. The auricular nerve, cited as being part of the facial nerve, is further to the back of the head, and can be worked by extending the SCM draining moves across the back of the mastoid. The temporal muscle works with the masseter to create a huge degree of tension and strain, as well as power for the jaw. It protects the thinnest part of the skull by means of muscle sinews that are like steel wires, often wrapped up in thick fascial bands, blended into the smooth curve of the skull in the zygomatic arch.

The whole sequence of moves, although seemingly complex, takes only a few seconds and creates an enormous release of tension and energy through the head. Further drainage along the length of the SCM can then take place, which may sometimes be performed three or four times for severe hay fever sufferers or others suffering from congestion.

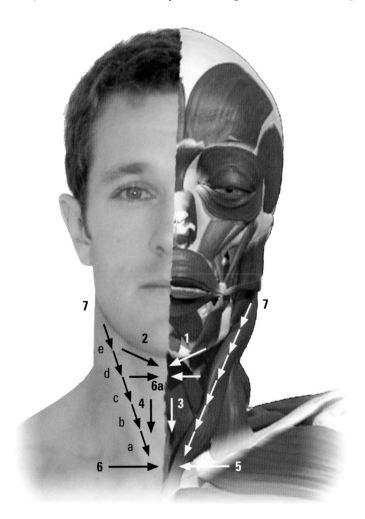

TMJ and hay fever.

VAGUS, THE WANDERER

The vagus nerve is the tenth and longest of the cranial nerves and its name gives a clue to its nature but less so to its function. The length and meandering nature of the nerve makes it a vagrant, wandering vaguely through the body and branching off several times into various organs and functions.

The vagus nerve is a nerve of the parasympathetic nervous system, the branch of the ANS which deals with the resting and digesting functions of the body. It is opposite in function to the sympathetic nervous system, but, in an ideal world, both these systems work in harmony and balance. The vagus nerve secretes a neurotransmitter – a chemical information carrier – called acetylcholine (ACh), which slows the heart rate down. A slow heart rate is very important for digestion: a high heart rate or stress after eating leads to very poor digestion, ulcers and heartburn – a case against fast food if ever there was one.

The vagus nerve passes through the neck on its way down and around the body, and is closest to the surface in the vicinity of the SCM. This is one reason why it is suggested that the coccyx and TMJ procedures not be performed in the same session, thus avoiding a conflict or confusion between the two systems of the ANS. In conclusion, the TMJ procedure is a major structural balancer of the body and will work very well with, for example, ankle and pelvis moves, to create a sound structural grounding.

CAUTION

Over the years I have seen many profound responses to TMJ work, and it is not uncommon for small changes in the bite to occur. In cases where a lot of dental work has been done, caution should be exercised; if in any doubt, the TMJ should not be performed. The drainage and SCM moves, however, can be safely administered in these instances.

Many people ask whether a disclaimer form can be filled in, whereby the client indemnifies the therapist if anything should go wrong. In the UK this form is legally not very sound, but apart from that, the therapist needs to follow their own instinct. If you have any concerns or worries about the effects of a particular procedure or treatment on an individual, then simply don't continue. Follow the hunch!

CHAPTER 19

Getting 'Them' Better: The Outcome Paradigm

One of the most challenging elements of any kind of therapy work is when clients don't respond to treatment that we are giving them. I say 'don't respond'; however, what I should emphasise is clients don't appear to respond. There is a world of difference between the non-responding client and the apparently non-responding client.

The first consideration is to summon closely what our own role or expectation is in the process of healing or changing a client. I am fond of stirring up a group of therapists by suggesting that it is not our job to get someone better. It is a controversial statement, but something which is useful to discuss, as we put a lot of store by our ability to heal, suggesting that we fail if we don't.

I would suggest, however, that there are only three possible outcomes to any therapeutic intervention:

1. The client gets better.

2. The client has no apparent change.

3. The client gets worse.

Anyone who has worked in bodywork for a period of time will have experienced all three of these outcomes. We of course have to hope that we have many more number ones than number twos or threes, but part of our learning experience will be those people who don't respond to the treatment we are offering. What is interesting is that if we look at our motivations or thought processes when we are treating these people, none of us will go into a treatment room with the intention of treating somebody in such a way that they get worse or don't change. Our natural desires as therapists are always to help people in pain.

The natural order of things means that not everyone we work with will respond in the way that perhaps we would like, or indeed they would like. We can, however, mitigate the number of non-responding clients by investigating areas in which perhaps we can improve ourselves. The starting point for this is to take on board the statement that a successful treatment is not dependent on the outcome. However good a therapist you are, there will be people who just don't get better, no matter what you do.

The first port of call when examining non-responding clients is to look at the quality and level of note-taking. I have devoted a whole chapter to this complex subject (see Chapter 21), but suffice to say that the effectiveness of our work will only be demonstrated by our notes. Inadequate notes will let us and the client down, prevent us from being able to evaluate effectively outcomes and changes, and significantly restrict our ability to feed back relevant changes to our clients.

The second step in examining our own role is to consider areas where perhaps we had not anticipated problems might lie. We can see from some of the other chapters that going straight to the region of pain is not always helpful or the answer to the problem. We will often need to consider other areas of the body that might be relevant, and we need to ask the client sufficient questions to establish a clear history and pattern of any given problem.

The next area we can consider is whether perhaps our treatment is appropriate in terms of whether we have done too much, not done enough, or generally not worked with combinations that might be more effective. A lot of this comes with experience, whilst as much of it is about guesswork and a degree of luck. Again, it is very hard to predict what is going to happen. Even after over 20 years of working with clients, I can never be sure about outcomes and am often surprised.

Once we have eliminated our own role in the reasons why the client is not progressing, we can start to look at whether the client has a role to play. Re-injury is a common component. Take, for example, a client who feels great right after the treatment but for whom this response does not last. Within three or four days they return to their original levels of pain and are naturally disappointed. Of course, we need to check that the functional levels are still the same, and if this kind of pattern happens more than two or three times, we need to establish that there has been no re-injury during the week. A re-injury can take several forms:

1. A conscious re-injury, where the client is fully aware that they have done something to themselves.

2. A subconscious re-injury, where the client has perhaps unwittingly performed an action or movement which has negated the effects of the treatment. Examples might be lifting a bin sharply, opening the curtains, being pulled by the dog when out walking, and wearing high heels. It is down to the therapist to try to establish this situation by observation and questioning.

3. A habitual postural re-injury, where the client is sitting, lying, driving, working or playing in a manner which is both creating the problem and re-emphasising it, even after treatment. Again, the therapist needs to get the relevant information out of the client by a system of questioning and observation.

Several years ago I had a client whom I had effectively given up on. The treatment didn't seem to last for more than three or four days, and whilst she felt many other benefits, the original lower-back problem kept on coming back time after time. I just couldn't get to the bottom of it. After about three months she returned, bringing her husband to the treatment session; she was sitting in the consultation room and made a little jump on her chair to bring it forwards. It seemed like an unusual action, and I commented on it to them both. "Oh, she always does that," said her husband. It was then that I realised it was this strange jumping action which was in fact causing an effective re-injury after each treatment. It had become such a habit with her that she hardly even realised she was doing it.

The car is a good example of a place where re-injuries are common. On more than one occasion I have gone and sat in a client's car to see if I could get a feel for what they were doing, or how they were sitting. Another thing to check is your client's shoes to see where they are worn down, and similarly look for any degree of callus build-up on their feet.

The last section about considering the role your client plays concerns a statement that I frequently hear from complementary therapists. They dismiss the client who is not responding effectively to treatment by saying: "Oh, they just don't want to get better." This is one statement that is guaranteed to annoy me. Who are we to decide that someone doesn't want to get better? I believe that everyone wants to achieve their full potential, be free of pain, and lead a happy and fulfilling life. The reality is that many people have learned patterns and ways of behaviour that might get in the way of them achieving this. My response to the 'they don't want to get better' statement, would be to suggest to the therapist that perhaps they themselves are not skilled or accomplished enough to recognise the steps that the client needs to take.

I do of course accept that there are certain situations where the timing and circumstances just aren't right. The steps that a client might need to put in place in order to change could be just too big or unattainable at this present moment. It might be that the interpersonal dynamics between the therapist and the client aren't right, or that there are other emotional issues that underlie the presentation. None of these represents a lack of desire for change on behalf of the client. I feel that it is our role as therapists to try to put ourselves in the mind and body of the client. We cannot drag anyone into a process of change, but instead need to understand what small steps an individual might be able to take.

After all these considerations, what we have to try to practise most of all is patience. We are not going to fix everyone. We are not going to achieve 100% success. I am of the firmly held belief that clients who don't respond or are difficult to work with and treat represent brilliant opportunities for us to learn. They are in essence our kind teachers. They make us examine ourselves, our knowledge, our practice, and confidence in what we do. Once we have done this, however, it is important to move on and not get stuck in the concept of failure.

Also vital is the need to examine our own expectations in relation to how we work with clients. How many of us, before we even start, have discussed what it is that the client would like to achieve from any sessions they have with us? Whereas our desire may be to have a particular client running up hills, they might just want to be able to sleep better, have a little bit more mobility, or even a slight reduction in pain. The mismatch of expectations is a recipe for disappointment. My grandfather had a wonderful phrase which, looking back, I realise is a teaching of mindfulness and an exhortation to rely on a happy mind. He said: "Blessed is he that expecteth nothing, for he shall not be disappointed."

CHAPTER 20

Reasons Why Bowen Works: Placebo Effect?

Bowen acknowledges the person as well as the pain or problem. The body is treated and respected as a whole, without reference to a named disease. Bowen understands the differences that each person presents. It is this art of listening and hearing which promotes trust and therefore repair. The role of the placebo effect cannot be overstated and should be relied on and trusted. It is a role that modern medicine should aspire to.

All medicine is a placebo to some degree; if it's not, then it should be. The word 'placebo' comes from the Latin, meaning 'I will please'. The first recorded medical reference to it was around 1785: "a medicine given more to please than to benefit the patient". It seems tautological: how can a medicine which pleases not have some benefit as well? Given that most medicine in 1785 was almost entirely useless, pretty much anything that didn't kill the patient could have been considered a bonus!

These days, the word 'placebo' is a stick used to beat complementary medicine and is considered a byword for 'useless'. Whilst I have no shame, worry or concern over the use of the word placebo when applied to Bowen, I am also entirely convinced that Bowen is not solely a placebo. The technique produces measurable changes and outcomes, and there is no doubt that these physiological changes come about as a direct result of the work done to the client by the therapist.

However, even pharmaceutical intervention has some degree of placebo attached to it. A pill might have a certain function, determined under laboratory conditions. But, in the hands of a doctor, the ability to enhance the power of the drug is greater if a compassionate, listening and caring environment is provided alongside the medication.

As Bowen therapists, we provide the opportunity for the client to express not just the physical symptoms that they are experiencing, but also how they might feel about these problems – how these affect them day to day, and how their lives might be altered or challenged. The changes we see may not be a complete restoration of function, but instead a gradual improvement in their quality of life: less pain rather than no pain, better sleep, a greater ability to relax and engage with the world around them, and less medication perhaps and therefore greater clarity of mind.

Hands-on treatments are no doubt effective, and we need to study as much as possible the reasons why we manage to achieve the changes that we do. Yet we must also remember the role we play, since a listening and understanding ear is sometimes as important as the procedures we use. The skill of listening also includes the skill of drawing out the information we need, editing what is being said, and keeping the session relevant and within the allotted time – all without being too rushed or direct!

Private Eye columnist Phil Hammond, who writes under the pseudonym MD, wrote an article criticising the decision of 13 senior consultants to write to *The Times* in May 2006, demanding that the NHS should stop funding alternative therapies. His argument was that "all medicine is in large part placebo, yet some doctors are jealous of the complementary therapists' freedom to 'big up' their placebo effect by talking unscientific bollocks".

He cites evidence that of all the thousands of conventional medical treatments reviewed by 'Clinical Evidence.com', only 15% have been shown to be of proven benefit. Given that a recent study of 1130 people receiving Bowen showed that 93% of them reported benefit, the difference could hardly be more striking.

Hammond is no apologist for complementary medicine and takes the lazy and easy view adopted by most medical professionals that most CAM is sham. But he does go on to make some interesting observations that put the placebo effect on the level of some very powerful drugs and concludes that the National Health Service would 'implode' without the input of complementary therapy.

A study which appeared in the Archives of General Psychiatry in 1965 reported on a group of 15 psychiatric patients who were offered a placebo drug and were even told what it was. In spite of knowing that it was a sugar pill, 14 of them agreed to give it a go and 13 improved – some a great deal.

In his book *13 Things That Don't Make Sense* (Profile Books, 2009), quantum physicist Michael Brooks discusses one of the most popular anti-anxiety drugs of the 20th century, diazepam, marketed under the trade name Valium by Hoffman LaRoche. A remarkable study showed that, simply put, diazepam doesn't work unless you know you're taking it, with the researchers suggesting that "anxiety reduction after open diazepam administration (people who knew they were taking it) was a placebo effect".

With such powerful effects, it's no wonder that drug companies struggle to beat the effects of placebos in human trials. But it also begs the question as to what we do when we consider treating whole persons and change the way they feel about themselves. Perhaps it is time to consider the placebo effect as a valuable part of human interaction and teach our doctors that old-fashioned 'bedside manners' really do matter.

CHAPTER 21

Effective Note-Taking: Client and Therapist Observation and Markers

There are two people involved in taking notes – the client and the therapist – both of whom need to contribute fully if the exercise is to be productive. There are also two types of information that can be gathered by the client and therapist:

1. Observations

2. Markers

By checking to see that all the areas are covered we will find that we have gathered some practical and useful information which will enable us to make effective week-to-week comparisons.

OBSERVATIONS

An observation is a comment made by the client or therapist which lacks a basis for measurement. It is useful information because it tells us how the client feels about themselves or their condition, but it doesn't give clear indications which can be measured during the following weeks.

CLIENT OBSERVATIONS

"I feel very stiff all over", "I feel old", "I'm in some sort of pain most of the time", "I don't get about like I used to", "My leg doesn't move very easily", "I'm quite tired and lethargic".

Although for each of these statements we could probe the client further to get more detail, the statements in themselves don't have a well-defined point from which we could take measurements. They are, however, still important, and we can go back to see if the client feels the same later, although it is harder to establish if there is any change. The usefulness of some observations can be enhanced by asking questions about what was said. For example, "I can't walk very far" could easily be turned into a marker (see below) by finding out how far the client can walk and why they have to stop.

THERAPIST OBSERVATIONS

The same principle as for client observations applies to anything that we observe about our client and for which we cannot get a defined measurement. If their jaw opens and closes strangely, or they have a certain way of walking or sitting, it might be difficult to describe this in writing. We can, however, make the observation as a reminder for us to check to see if anything has changed by the time the next treatment comes along.

Observations don't necessarily relate to something that we think might be wrong with a client: they could be particulars that catch our eye, and may or may not be relevant. By practising the art of looking at things and making observations, we will be drawn to asking questions and building the skill of intuitive bodywork, which is the essence of the Bowen Technique.

MARKERS

A marker is a point which provides a clear reference for comparison purposes. Markers are generally not going to be volunteered by the client and instead will come from asking specific questions. For instance, a client might say that they have difficulty walking up the stairs; by questioning them further we can find out how many stairs they can climb before they need to rest. Another client might say that they can't walk very far. Again, by continuing a little bit further, we might ascertain that they can walk up to the end of the road to the post office, before they have to turn around and come home. This gives us a clear marker from which to measure changes from week to week.

A lot of the time the changes with Bowen will be very subtle, and it will be only the notes that will clearly reflect what is different. Markers give us control over the information we obtain and are the most effective way of reflecting change. We should aim for at least four client markers in each session. Photographs are also an excellent way to set markers and provide evidence that is irrefutable.

THERAPIST MARKERS

Therapist markers are again specific and only obtainable through measurements. We can say that the client appears to be very stiff in the way they move their shoulders, which would be a therapist observation. Or we can see that they are in pain and struggle when putting on a jacket or coat. We can then create markers using measurements, such as the percentage of movement, but only if we have established a base point for what 'zero' corresponds to.

Pain scales can also be used, but only in addition to other information – they should not be used exclusively as markers. Any pain scales used should be explained to the client, indicating what level '0' is and what '10' would be. However, these scales are not always very reliable; although they can be a useful tool, they should only form a small part of the way you gather effective information. If you want to measure ranges of movement, again set a baseline from which to start. You might draw a stick man, use a comparison with a clock face or employ a measuring instrument such as a goniometer.

Other markers can come from checking the level of medication that a client is taking. If, for example, they are taking eight painkillers a day, we can check in weeks two and three to see if this has changed.

Other medications, such as sleeping tablets or asthma medication, might also have changed, although we do need to make sure that we are not encouraging our clients to stop taking medication.

BODY OUTLINES

A body outline sheet is a very useful tool that serves to illustrate the written notes very well. Clients will often forget other areas where pain problems present, and such a sheet will remind them. Working with the client, we can go through the body outline briefly, from top to bottom, and covering the back and the front, noting areas where there are clear problems or pain. If you determine an area where there is an issue or condition, shade it, date it and give a brief description. You can go back to this in later treatments to check whether the problem has shifted, or even to see if there is a different problem somewhere else.

If there are multiple presentations and the client has a lot of issues, write down a problem list and ask the client to prioritise the complaints. It is often the case that the therapist makes the decision as to what should be treated, and yet, by asking the client, this view might easily change.

WHY DO WE NEED TO MAKE NOTES?

Many people assume that notes aren't always that important. The subtle nature of Bowen, however, means that in many cases clients will come back for a second or third treatment, with little idea what, if anything, has changed. If you as the therapist are unable to tell them, it will appear that nothing has happened.

The majority of clients don't give you all the relevant information. It is not because they want to mislead you, but simply because they have forgotten or haven't been asked the right questions. Sufficient detail in your notes gives leads that will unlock this closed-off information by enabling you to ask a wider range of questions and therefore have a greater chance of gathering all the necessary details. This in turn will make your treatment more effective.

The third area relates to the law: it is important to establish what has been said and done in any given treatment session, in case there is any suggestion that you have not acted properly. In this instance your notes become a legal record of what has happened. Although notes can't record everything said, plenty of written information will give a good feel to the content of the session.

QUESTIONNAIRES

A lot of existing therapists ask their clients to fill out standard questionnaire forms. These can range in complexity from simple name and address and contact details, to complex previous medical history, medication, surgery, whether your mother was left-handed, and so forth. Personally I find these questionnaires somewhat pointless, although I can see the benefit in some situations. I prefer to start with a blank sheet of paper and listen carefully to what the client is saying and how they are saying it. From the basic information that I receive, I will subsequently raise serious questions and draw out measurable and quantifiable markers.

I cannot tell you the number of times that clients have returned with a certain view of how the treatment is progressing, only to be somewhat better informed once they've been properly appraised of their progress over a period of weeks. Taking notes is an art in itself and one of the single most important elements in a clinical environment. However good you think you are as a therapist, the only proof you have lies in the notes you take: everything else is conjecture.

TYPES OF QUESTION TO ASK

PAIN / SORENESS / COMPLAINT

Where is it?

What type of pain is it: stabbing, aching, shooting?

How long have you had it?

Is it there all the time?

Do you feel it at the moment?

When do you notice it the most?

If your level of pain is scored from 1 to 10, with 10 being absolute agony and 1 being hardly anything, what is the average?

Does it wake you up in the night? How many nights a week?

What does it stop you from doing?

Does it spread to other areas?

RESTRICTION / STIFFNESS

How much stiffness?

What is the restriction?

If a measurement is required, where is it from and to? In other words, what is the normal movement and what is the restriction compared to that?

What kind of activity does the restriction or stiffness prevent?

STRESS

What is the source of stress: job, relationship, children, money?

What exactly is stressful about the specific source of stress?

What does stress mean to you?

Do you always feel like this?

LOW ENERGY / TIRED

How tired are you?

Do you sleep well? If so, what do you mean by 'well': how many hours?

What happens when you get tired?

When do you get tired?

What do you do when you get tired?

Does anything help your energy levels?

Is there anything you do that causes you to feel your energy coming back?

SUBSEQUENT TREATMENTS

The treatment follow-up is all-important in subsequent weeks. Don't rely on the client to give you reliable feedback – they will often have forgotten what the problem was or the severity and nature of it. This means that your notes from the first week must be a good record. If they are, then you just need to go back to them to compare. If you decide that no treatment is needed in week two, or in subsequent weeks, then simply don't treat the client, but nevertheless record your decisions and reasons.

Following up your client after the treatment is a good idea. I ask clients to return after a period of four weeks from the last treatment, and will then suggest that they return every six to eight weeks to keep topped up and prevent further problems from arising. If you take this approach, there are many ways of managing and servicing your clients: this will be the subject of a future book.

CHAPTER 22

Conclusion

The UK has recently seen a spate of complaints to the Advertising Standards Authority (ASA) from people challenging the claims made by various practitioners of complementary therapy, Bowen included. Whilst we have already talked about the need to avoid claims being made, the need to discuss the remarkable results that we achieve will naturally see us in conflict with those who feel that anything that is not 'mainstream' should be restricted.

The United Kingdom allows the freedom to practise CAM – a freedom virtually unknown to most of the rest of the world. As practitioners, we do not have to be registered, be approved of, sit exams or take continuing development courses. We are not regulated or inspected, and can treat anyone with anything. The difference is that we shouldn't be treating conditions, nor claim that we can, unless we have specific results from properly conducted research. A case in point is the hamstring research mentioned earlier, which allows Bowen therapists to quite freely state that a single treatment of the Bowen Technique significantly increases hamstring flexibility.

It is inevitable that more issues will arise where people will complain about the lack of effective research into our technique. We know it works, we know we get incredibly good results and we know that something is going on in the body that perhaps we will never be able to explain. The responsibility lies with our own community to undertake more in the way of research. But research is expensive and time consuming. Publishing the results is also difficult, but these factors should not deter us; joint efforts from the various schools and associations need to be put in place. The politics of envy has seen that peer-reviewed research is not even referred to by certain sections of the Bowen community, and sometimes other studies are lauded, even though they are of poor quality and design.

In ten years' time the face of health will continue to change as an elderly population seeks answers from an increasingly cash-strapped government. Prevention needs to be embraced as a major tool in the health systems of the world. The mentality that we can sit and wait for pain and imbalances to show up before treating them leads purely to expensive and ineffective treatment methods. The paradigm of reductionist anatomy will also need to be addressed if medicine is going to understand more of both how the body moves and the relationships that exist through our various systems. None of these transitions will happen quickly, and progress is often seen as a procession of funerals, with people quite literally waiting for obstructions and objections to be carried away before moving to a productive and constructive place.

For me Bowen continues to be my life work. I see no merit in extending it, changing its name or principles, or messing around with the past. The technique's validity rests on the solidity of its consistent outcomes over the last 30 years. Whilst I fully accept the need to scrutinise, study and test its methods, I see no reason why it should not continue to grow and be more widely accepted and available.

RESOURCES

Bell, M.A. and Fox, N.A. (1997). 'Individual differences in object permanence performance at 8 months: Locomotor experience and brain electrical activity', *Developmental Psychobiology* 31(4): 287–297.

Biel, A. (2005). *The Trail Guide to the Body*. Boulder, CO: Books of Discovery.

ClinicalEvidence (2012). Website: www.clinicalevidence.com.

Dadebo, B., White, J. and George, K.P. (2004). A survey of flexibility training protocols and hamstring strains in professional football clubs in England. *Br. J. Sports Med.*, 38: 338-394.

Drake, R.L., Vogl, A.W. and Mitchell, A.W.M. (2010). *Gray's Anatomy for Students*. Philadelphia: Churchill Livingstone/Elsevier.

Falvey, E.C., Clark, R.A., Franklyn-Miller, A. et al. (2010). 'Iliotibial band syndrome: An examination of the evidence behind a number of treatment options', *Scand J Med Sci Sports* 20(4): 580–587.

Gabbe, B.J., Finch, D.F., Bennell, K.L. and Wajsweiner. (2005). Risk factors for hamstring injuries in community level Australian football. *Br. J. Sports Med.*, 39: 106-110.

Gleim, G.W. and McHugh, M.P. ((1997). Flexibility and its effects on sports injury and performance. *Sp. Med.* 24(5), 289-299.

Hayashi, M., Motoyoshi, N. and Hori, T. (2005). 'Recuperative power of a short daytime nap with or without stage 2 sleep', *Sleep* 28(7): 829–836.

Hedley, G. (2007). *The Integral Anatomy Series* (Integral Anatomy Productions, LLC) [DVD].

Hoskins, W.T. and Pollard, H.P. (2005). Successful management of hamstring injuries in Australian rules footballers: two case studies. *Chiropr. Osteopath*, 13: 4.

Juhan, D. (2003). *Job's Body*. New York: Barrytown/Station Hill.

Kershaw, E.E. and Flier, J.S. (2004). 'Adipose tissue as an endocrine organ', *J Clin Endocrinol Metab* 89(6): 2548–2556.

Langevin, H.M. and Sherman, K.J. (2006). Pathophysical model for chronic low back pain integrating connective tissue and nervous system mechanisms. *Medical Hypotheses,* Elsevier.

Levine, P.A. (1997). *Waking the Tiger: Healing Trauma Through the Body.* Berkeley, CA: North Atlantic Books.

Marr, M., Baker, J., Lambon, N. and Perry, J. (2011). 'The effects of the Bowen technique on hamstring flexibility over time: A randomised controlled trial', *J Bodywork Mov Ther* 15(3): 281–290.

Marwan, F. Abu-Hijleh and Harris, P.F. (2009). 'Extensor retinacular of the ankle and foot: Do they exist as illustrated in textbooks?', *Proc 2nd Intl Fascia Research Congress* (Amsterdam) 2: 324.

Moore, W. (2006). *The Knife Man.* London: Bantam.

Moseley, J.B., O'Malley, K., Petersen, N.J. et al. (2002). 'A controlled trial of arthroscopic surgery for osteoarthritis of the knee', *New England J Med* 347:81–88.

Murphy, D.R. (1991). A critical look at static stretching: are we doing our patients harm? *Chiroprac. Sp. Med.,* 5(3), 67-70.

Murray, C. (2010). *In Search of Tom Bowen.* Ringwood Vic, Australia: Palmer Higgs.

NICE (2009). 'Early management of persistent non-specific low back pain' (Clinical Guidelines CG88, May).

Oschman, J.L. (2000). *Energy Medicine: The Scientific Basis.* Edinburgh: Churchill Livingstone.

Park, L. and Covi, L. (1965). 'Non blind placebo trial', *Arch Gen Psych* 12: 336–345.

Pischinger, A. (2007). *The Extracellular Matrix and Ground Regulation: Basis for a Holistic Biological Medicine.* Berkeley, CA: North Atlantic Books.

Sapolsky, R. (2004). *Why Zebras Don't Get Ulcers.* New York: Holt.

Saunders, J.B. de C.M. and O'Malley, C.D. (1950). *The Illustrations from the Works of Andreas Vesalius of Brussels.* Cleveland & New York: World Publishing Co.

Schleip, R. (2012). Fascia: The Tensional Network of the Human Body: *The Science and Clinical Applications in Manual and Movement Therapy.* Elsevier, London.

Saal, J. S. (1987). Flexibility training in physical medicine and rehabilitation. State of Art Reviews, 1(4), 537-554.

Shyne, K. and Dominguez, R. (1982). To stretch or not to stretch? *Physician and Sports Med.* 10, 137-140.

Vleeming, A., Pool-Goudzwaard, A., Hammudoghlu. D., Stoeckart, R., Snijders, C.J. and Mens, J.M. (1996). The function of the long dorsal sacroiliac ligament: its implication for understanding low back pain. *Spine,* 21:556–562

INDEX

Abcess, 86
Abdomen, 14, 86
Acetylcholine (ACh), 146
Achilles tendon, 66, 110
Acromion, 53
Acupuncture, 30
Adductor longus, 118, 119
Adipose tissue, 11, 12, 24, 33, 35, 38
Adrenal glands, 104
Adrenalin, 74
Aerodynamics, 24
Ageing process, 23
Anatomy, 17; trains, 17, 18
Angina, 86
Ankle, 47, 63
Anterior compartment, 108
Anterior superior iliac spine (ASIS), 121, 122
Anterior tibial fasciitis, 65
Appendix, 70
Appetite, regulation, 12
Appropriate response mechanism, 39
Areolar, 12
Arm, 86
Aspartame, 106
Asthma, 83–85
Athletes, 42
Atrophy, 15
Autonomic nervous system, 33, 74, 76, 78

Back pain, 14, 23, 42, 88
Bad breath, 106
Basic relaxation move, 45

Bedwetting, 80
Beetroot, 106
Beeturia, 106
Betacyanin, 106
Betaine, 106
Biceps femoris, 48, 96
Blockers, 27, 45
Blood, 11, 12; pressure, 104
Body, brushing, 69; outlines, 155
Bone, 11, 22
Boron, 106
Bowen move, 33, 35
Bowen, Tom, 25
Brachial plexus, 89, 143
Breakdown, 86
Breaks, 27, 29, 38
Breast, 69; cancer, 69; feeding, 69; implants, 72
Bronchodilator, 85

Cancer, 106
Callus, 149
Capillaries, 34
Carpal tunnel syndrome, 90, 93, 132
Cartilage, 11
Cellulose, 15, 23
Central nervous system, 12
Cervical spine, 143
Chest, 86; pains, 84
Childbirth, 75
Chronic obstructive pulmonary disease, 83
Circulatory system, 70, 71
Clavicle, 132

Claw toes, 65
Coccyx, 69, 73, 74, 79, 113, 124, 146
Colic, 84
Collagen, 15, 23, 108
Colon, 76
Common peroneal nerve, 99
Conclusion, 159
Connective tissue, 11
Cornea, 15
Corticosterone, 104
Cortisol, 104
Coventry university, 97
Cranberries, 106
Cytokines, 12

Dairy, 84
Dehydroepiandrosterone, 104
Deltoid, 51, 52, 69, 91, 129, 132
Diaphragm, 71, 79, 81–83, 85, 117; move, 37
Dorsal spine, 81

Eczema, 76, 84
Elasticity, 34
Elbow, 89
Emergency move, 85
Emotional, 78
Endocrine, 12
Energetic strain, 87
Energy, 46
Erector spinae, 37, 46, 53, 55
Erythema, 34, 46
European College of Bowen Studies (ECBS),
    97, 117, 118
Exhalation, 37
Extensor digitorum communis, 91
Extensor digitorum longus, 64
Extensor retinaculum, 63, 92
Eyeball pressure, 34

Fascia, 11, 15, 18, 22, 41; connections, 22;
    superficial, 11, 12, 23, 33, 35
Feed-forward mechanism, 124
Femur, 113
Fibril, 23
Fibroblast, 15

Fibularis, brevis, 65; longus, 65
Fight-or-flight response, 74, 104
Five-minute break, 101
Flat feet, 65
Flexor digitorum longus, 65
Fluid dynamics, 24
Foot, 63
Frozen shoulder, 52, 132

Galea aponeurotica, 142
Galen, 19
Gall bladder, 86
Ganglion impar, 78
Gastrocnemius, 110
Gluteal muscles, 47
Gluteus maximus, 13, 47, 52
Gracilis, 119, 120
Gray, Henry, 20
Greater occipital nerve, 58
Growth, 86

Hamstring, 47, 95, 107; flexibility, 41
Harvey, William, 19
Hay fever, 145
Head, 57
Heart, 81
Heat, 13
Hedley, Gill, 21, 117
Hip bone, 113
Hit the lat (HTL), 48, 67, 101, 109, 110, 118
Holding point, 78
Holistic, 23
Homogenisation, 84
Hooke's law, 24
Hormones, 69, 104
Humerus, 54
Hunter, John, 20

Iliacus, 121
Iliotibial band, 21, 22, 37, 48, 64, 97, 108, 122;
    syndrome, 108
Ilium, 121
Imbalances, 23
Immune system, 12
Indigestion, 85

Inflammation, 12
Infraspinatus, 130
Inguinal ligament, 121
Insulin, resistance, 12
Ischial tuberosity, 48, 96

Kidney, 71, 103; stones, 106
Kinesiology, 30
Knee, 47, 64, 71, 100, 107
Kyphosis, 85

Ladybirds, 53
Lateral epicondyle, 90
Latissimus dorsi, 52, 54
Leg-length difference, 115
Leg lock, 87
Leptin, 12
Levator scapulae, 51, 53, 58, 130
Libido, 74
Ligaments, 21
Light touch therapy, 34
Liposuction, 13
Liver, 82, 86
Lordosis, 85
Low energy, 157
Lower-back pain, 47, 98; problem, 148
Lung, 86
Lymphatic, 70, 117; drainage, 71, 82; tissues, 69; treatment, 54
Lymph nodes, 54, 71
Lymphoid organs, 70

Malleolus, 110
Markers, 153
Mastectomies, 72
Mastoid process, 141
Mechanoreceptors, 24
Medial epicondylitis, 90
Medial malleolus, 65
Median nerve, 89, 92
Meniscus, 108
Menstruation, 69
Mental, 78
Meridian, 30
Metabolism, regulation, 12

Metatarsal joints, 100
Milk, 84
Miscarriage, 79
Movement, 18, 23
Moves, 27, 29; direction, 37
Multifidus, 96
Muscle, 13, 21
Musculoskeletal, 75
Myers, Tom, 17

Navel, 14
Neck, 86; pain, 52; stretch, 137
Neurotransmitter, 146
Newton's law, 46
NICE, 14
Note-taking, 42, 148, 153

Obesity, 12
Observations, 153
Occipital, protuberance, 58; ridge, 58
Oestrogen, 104
Organic, 75
Oschman, James, 46
Ossification, 15
Outcome paradigm, 147

Page one, 37, 45, 60, 67, 118
Page three, 57, 60, 90
Page two, 37, 51, 60, 90, 109, 130
Pain, 42
Palliative care, 42
Palpation, 64
Parasympathetic nervous system, 74, 80, 146
Parietal peritoneum, 81, 83, 117
Pasteurisation, 84
Patella, 109
Patellar ligament, 109
Patience, 42
Pectoralis, 70, 131
Pelvic, floor, 74, 75, 77, 113; imbalance, 114; tilt, 114; triangle, 120
Pelvis, 47, 52, 71, 113
Pericardium, 81
Periosteum, 23, 64
Perirenal fat, 104

Peritoneal bag, 79
Phrenic nerve, 86
Piezoelectricity, 24
Placebo effect, 151
Plantar, fascia, 110;fasciitis, 112; flexion, 65
Plaque, 106
Plastic surgery, 13
Polyphenol antioxidants, 106
Popliteal fossa, 48, 71
Postural adjustment, 115
Posture, 15, 18, 23
Pregnancy, 79
Pressure, 33, 38
Primary motor complex, 40
Protein, 15, 23
Psoas muscle, 120
Psoriasis, 76
Pubic bone, 76, 118, 144

Qi, 46
Quadratus lumborum, 81, 88
Quadriceps femoris, 109
Questionnaires, 155

Radial nerve, 89
Radiohumeral joint, 92
Recoil, 24
Rectus abdominis, 76
Reductionist, 46
Re-injury, 148
Repetitive strain injury, 89, 94
Reproductive, 75
Resistin, 12
Respiration, 58, 70, 81
Respiratory dysfunction, 132, 143
Restriction, 156
Resurrectionists, 20
Rhomboids, 53
Rolling-type move, 33, 35
Rotator cuff, 23, 129
Russell, John Scott, 23

Sacroiliac, joint, 123; ligament, 46, 96, 123
Sacrotuberous ligament, 48, 96, 123
Sacrum, 46, 47, 63, 75, 113, 124

Sartorius, 120, 121
Scalenes, 58, 86
Scapula, 52, 70; winging, 52
Sciatica, 100
Sciatic nerve, 99, 112
Scoliosis, 85
Semispinalis capitis, 58
Semitendinosus, 48
Serratus anterior, 70
Shin splints, 65
Shoulder, 71, 86, 129; blade, 57; exercises, 135; girdle, 130, 133; procedure, 69
Skeleton, 21
Skin, 11, 33; slack, 33, 35, 36, 54, 58, 85
Sleep, 40
Snake movement, 92
Sock, 64
Soleus, 65, 110
Soliton waves, 23
Spinal column, 75
Spinalis capitis, 58
Spinal root nerves, 55
Spirals, 23
Spleen, 70
Splenius capitis, 59, 141
Stabilisers, 98
Sternocleidomastoid, 59, 140, 141; drainage, 140
Sternum, 85
Stiffness, 156
Stoppers, 29, 45, 46, 74
Stress, 73, 76, 104, 156
Stretching, 95
Stretch reflex, 95
Submandibular gland, 143
Superficial back line, 99
Supraspinatus, 53
Sympathetic chain, 78
Sympathetic nervous system, 74, 76
Synovial joint, 96

Temporal, bone, 59; muscle, 145
Temporomandibular joint, 59, 71, 134, 139; procedure, 80, 144
Tendon, 11, 21

Tennis elbow, 89
Tenosynovitis, 143
Teres major, 54, 133; minor, 54, 133
Testosterone, 104
Thoracolumbar fascia, 46, 54, 79, 96, 117, 125
Thymus, 70
Tibialis, anterior, 64; posterior, 65
Tibial nerve, 99
Tibiocalcaneal ligament, 65
Tibionavicular ligament, 65
Tibiotalar ligament, 65
Tired, 157
Tonsils, 70
Trachea, 144
Training course, 30
Transversus abdominis, 81, 83, 117
Trapezius, 51, 53, 58, 59, 130
Treatments, time between, 41; 157
Triple helix, 23
Twenty-eight (28) day rule, 134

Ulnar nerve, 89, 92
Urinary tract infections, 104

Vagina, 75
Vagus nerve, 145, 146
Vastus intermedius, 109
Vastus lateralis, 48, 109
Vesalius, 19
Viscera, 79, 117

Wave of translation, 23
Whiplash, 42
Whole-body treatment, 35

Xiphoid process, 85, 87

Zygomatic process, 144

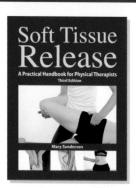
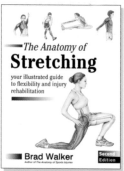
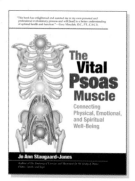
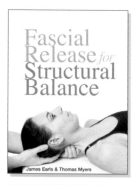
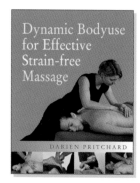
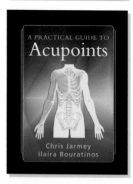
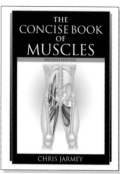
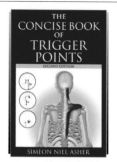
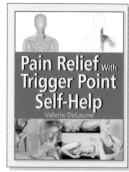